LOSE TEN POUNDS
in just <u>30</u> days

Neil Taylor

OLIVER
NELSON

THOMAS NELSON PUBLISHERS
Nashville

To

Larry and Rayna Bertolucci, whose renewed
physical fitness and positive attitudes are a lasting
source of inspiration.

Published in Nashville, Tennessee, by Oliver-Nelson Books, a division of
Thomas Nelson, Inc., Publishers, and distributed in Canada by Word
Communications, Ltd., Richmond, British Columbia.

The Bible version used in this publication is THE NEW KING JAMES
VERSION. Copyright © 1979, 1980, 1982, Thomas Nelson, Inc.,
Publishers.

Printed in the United States of America.

Library of Congress Cataloging-in-Publication Data

Taylor, Neil.
    How to lose ten pounds / Neil Taylor.
      p.   cm.
    ISBN 0-8407-9246-8 (pbk.)
    1. Reducing. I. Title.
RM222.2.T37   1993
613.2′5—dc20   93-4982
                                    CIP

1 2 3 4 5 6 — 98 97 96 95 94 93

CONTENTS

INTRODUCTION

This thirty-day plan for losing just ten pounds is not your typical diet and exercise program. In fact, it does not prescribe a particular program. Rather, it is a guided adventure in self-discovery, helping you find *your way* to become (and stay) ten pounds thinner. There are numerous ways to lose ten pounds. This book will help you find the way that works for you because you start where you are and make changes you can live with.

You can choose to lose ten pounds by choosing to change your lifestyle. Losing ten pounds is the effect you want to achieve; however, it is not truly your goal. In order to achieve the effect of weighing less while remaining healthy, your goals must include: eating a healthy selection of less fattening foods, enjoying activities that use up more of your body's energy reserves (i.e., fat), and changing your mind-set in ways that support your thinner self-image.

In the next thirty days you can change all of these things: your eating habits, your activity level, and your mind-set. When you do, you will gain a greater sense of self-confidence to go along with your more attractive physical appearance.

Most weight-loss programs tend to be negative. Our minds recoil at the thought of losing things. Even the term *weight loss* puts the focus on what you lose. Perhaps this has something to do with why dieting can be so intimidating.

Lose ten pounds and gain a healthier lifestyle.

This book is not about loss. With this plan you will focus on what you gain by living in more healthy ways. This book is about gaining the good things in life: a positive self-image, a healthier body, a renewed energy and zest for life, new strength, added self-confidence, a more attractive appearance, and increased comfort in social settings (not to mention greater comfort fitting into your jeans!). By gaining these positive attributes and healthful habits, you will not experience a sense of loss, even though you weigh ten pounds less.

D A Y

1

Finding Support

To lose weight and keep it off, you need support from those close to you. Changing your lifestyle to help you lose weight will affect the people around you, and those people will affect your efforts to lose weight. Therefore, it is important that you find consistent support from the very beginning.

From previous experience, you probably already know who will support you in losing weight and who will work against you. You could spend a great deal of time trying to figure out why some friends, family members, and loved ones seem intent on sabotaging your weight-loss efforts. However, even if you could figure out the reasons, you probably would not be able to change their attitudes or behavior toward you.

Therefore, for your purposes during the next thirty days, focus your attention on cultivating people who will support you.

———————————•———————————

Cultivate a support person for this adventure.

First, consider those who live with you. Since you will be changing the way you eat, shop for groceries, and cook, the best support you could get would be from those in your household. Since this is not your typical prescribed, restrictive diet plan, you may find that other family members are willing to explore finding a healthier way of life with you. Be sure to present this thirty-day period as a time of self-exploration and education to help each person find a less fattening way of life. You would have the best advantage if you could persuade all the members of your household to change your eating habits together. If this isn't going to work, try to find one other person in your home to join you.

If you live alone or don't find a supportive partner in your household, seek out a friend who would also like to lose ten pounds. By comparing notes you will be able to encourage each other, talk about things you are learning, and share the insights that are helping you change to a less fattening lifestyle.

If you are unable to find someone who also wants a new, thinner image, or if you would rather lose ten pounds on your own, find someone to support you for the next thirty days. A support person doesn't have to go the paces with you. Picture a long-distance runner who has support personnel driving alongside in a car. The runner goes through the paces on her own, but she has arranged to have a support team available whenever she shows signs of need. During these thirty days you will have moments when an encouraging voice, a proud smile, a nod of approval, or someone with whom to talk things over will prove extremely valuable.

Personal Evaluation

- Who among your circle of family, friends, and loved ones has demonstrated previous support of your attempts to lose excess weight?
- Are you willing to present this thirty-day plan to the members of your household in hopes of gaining a healthier lifestyle together?
- Name three people with whom you would enjoy following this plan or from whom you would like to receive support during the next thirty days.
- Think of someone you know who already lives a healthier lifestyle and who might be willing to offer you support.

Action

1. Talk to the members of your household and see if they would like to join you in exploring a healthier way of life together.

2. Contact the persons you have in mind to be your companions and ask them to join you.
3. If you don't want to or can't find a companion, find someone who will encourage you when you need support along the way.

Encouragement

By finding someone who will share your desire for a healthier lifestyle, you will make the adventure more fun and easier on yourself—especially if you work together to help each of you establish a new way of life.

Food for Thought

"Two are better than one, because they have a good reward for their labor. For if they fall, one will lift up his companion. But woe to him who is alone when he falls, for he has no one to help him up."

—Ecclesiastes 4:9–10

DAY 2

Starting Where You Are

You are a rare person indeed if this is the first time you have set out to lose weight. Dieting has become a national pastime. That Americans spent more than $35 billion on diet plans and supplements in 1990 is evidence of this fact. However, studies show that most people who lose weight by following a prescribed diet usually regain the weight (and then some) shortly after they stop dieting.

This book does not give you a prescribed diet plan to follow. Rather, it will help you to design an adapted lifestyle that will allow you to lose ten pounds and live at the lower weight you desire.

Many factors can contribute to gaining or losing weight. These include what you eat, when you eat, where you eat, how you eat, whether you have an eating disorder, your emotional relationship to food, your schedule, your level of physical activity, your self-image, your knowledge about nutrition, and your beliefs about what constitutes a healthy lifestyle.

In order to lose ten pounds, you must begin where you are. Assess the factors that contribute to your carrying around extra weight; then make changes that address these factors in your particular lifestyle.

When you evaluate your lifestyle, don't focus your attention on where you may be "bad" or "good." Focus on being accurate in terms of what you really do, believe, and want. In any endeavor, the key to successful change is to take an accurate measurement of the current situation.

Following are the areas in which you will be taking inventory of your current way of life.

Your Physical Activity

In this age of labor-saving devices, you may assume that you move around much more than you actually do. The fact that you accomplish a great deal from day to day doesn't necessarily mean that you have expended physical energy. The fact that you feel fatigue at the end of the day doesn't mean that your body is tired from physical activity. You may actually feel fatigue from a lack of physical activity. You need to become aware of how much physical movement and activity you get each day.

Eating Habits

To a large extent, your eating habits determine the weight at which you remain. You are trying to become aware of your eating habits so that you can choose which, if any, of these habits you want to change.

Your Emotional Relationship to Food

Look for the connection between your emotional feelings and your eating habits. Whenever you eat, ask yourself if you were physically hungry, if there was an emotional trigger to your decision to eat, or if there was an emotional hunger you were trying to satisfy. Examples of an emotional trigger might be feeling guilty over leaving food on your plate or feeling deprived of something and telling yourself, "I deserve a treat." Feelings of loneliness, grief, sadness, boredom, guilt, fear, and anger often act as triggers.

You may also eat whenever you are trying *not* to feel something. You may be inclined to stuff down feelings you want to avoid by stuffing yourself with food. Whenever you eat, try to notice whether you are physically hungry or whether there is an emotional attachment to your desire to eat.

Eating Disorders

There are several eating disorders. The three most commonly noted include compulsive overeating (typically, eating for emotional reasons or binging after periods of deprivation); bulimia (overeating and binging on large amounts of food, then using vomiting or laxatives to purge the food from the body); and anorexia (physically starving your body, and sometimes compulsively exercising, in an attempt to lose weight when you are actually under a healthy weight).

Schedule

Your schedule can have a direct effect on your weight. If your work is sedentary and requires a majority of your waking hours, you may have to make an extra effort to incorporate physical activity into your daily life. If you travel a lot, you will need to evaluate how you can adapt your eating and activities on the go. If you are overcommitted and don't plan your meals carefully, your reliance on convenience foods and fast foods may have a big impact on your weight.

Personal Evaluation

- What do you do in terms of physical activity on a daily basis?
- Check to see if your eating patterns may involve an eating disorder. Since persons having these disorders sometimes also have problems with denial, ask someone who knows you well to give input regarding whether you may be dealing with an eating disorder. If you suspect that this may be the case, seek help from a qualified professional.
- Keep track of your schedule, especially noting how eating fits in to what you do each day.
- In what way do the demands of your current schedule and commitments influence when you eat, what you eat, and where you eat?

Action

1. Create a notebook to use for recording your experiences and insights during this adventure.

   Today you will focus your attention on noting your current level of physical activity. On following days you will monitor other aspects of your behavior. Jot down a record of what physical movements your body experiences today. Across the top of a sheet of paper, write the following headings: *When, What Motion, Where, Why, Emotional Feelings,* and *Physical Feelings.*

2. Use each column to keep track of when you move. (You probably won't want to stop to do this after each move. Perhaps you can take time every few hours to keep track of what physical motion your body goes through. A possible schedule might be: mid-morning, before lunch, mid-afternoon, before dinner, mid-evening, and before bed.) Use the following guidelines for each column.

- when (note the time involved as precisely as possible)
- what (record anything you did: from sitting at a desk typing to working out at aerobics class)
- where (note movements to and from, such as: walked to car, drove, walked into office, stood in elevator, walked to desk, sat down)
- why (your purpose in moving could be functional—to get to work; emotional—for fun, to work off anger; or purposeful—to get an aerobic workout)
- emotional feelings (how you felt about doing the activity, such as: OK, good, bad, great, and so on)

- physical feelings (how your body felt while doing the activity, such as: tense, relaxed, energized, stiff, sore, and so on)

3. After you have tracked an actual day's activity, estimate your typical workday and a typical day off or weekend day's activity, using the same column headings. Later you can use these estimates of your activity level to help you choose when and how to become somewhat more active in ways that fit your lifestyle.

Encouragement

Getting an accurate reading of your physical activity level should not become evidence used to condemn yourself. Rather, congratulate yourself on facing reality so that you can actively move toward a healthier lifestyle.

Food for Thought

"If you can't measure it, you can't control it."
—John W. Hartley

DAY

3

Just Say No to Dieting and Deprivation

The latest research may validate what you already know from experience. Dieting doesn't usually help people lose weight and keep it off. Rather, what is lost through restrictive dieting, calorie counting, and self-enforced hunger is quickly regained once you stop dieting.

There is a logical explanation for this tendency to regain as much as or more than is lost during dieting. If you are severely restricting your body's intake of nourishing food, your body has no way to tell the difference between a self-imposed lack of food and starvation. When your body senses you are not getting what you need, the physical reaction is to slow down your metabolism so your energy reserves (i.e., stores of fat) are burned at a slower pace. If there were a true shortage of food, this would prolong survival. However, when the food shortage is self-imposed, the only thing prolonged is the time it will take for you to burn off fat.

———————●———————

Dieters often find themselves in a repetitious cycle.

———————————

Many people go through a season of life without ever thinking about weight control. But once they begin dieting, they find themselves caught in a repetitious cycle. The cycle may start when some change occurs in the body chemistry that results in a noticeable weight gain. The most common examples are puberty, pregnancy, menopause, or a change in lifestyle such as getting married or moving away to college.

In reaction to the weight gain, many persons decide to diet, artificially restricting what is eaten. The body experiences hunger, and its craving for nutritious foods is ignored. This can set up a cycle in which the body's physical cravings increase, eventually causing the dieter to "give in" and eat ravenously. Along with this, the metabolism may slow down to make sure there are extra reserves in case of any other unanticipated periods of hunger.

This cycle of dieting and overeating results in an ongoing weight problem. If you are one who has been caught up in trying one diet after another, only to regain your excess weight, this may explain how you ended up at war with your appetite. However, perhaps you can remember a time before you started dieting when you were more in tune with your body, when you ate when you were hungry and maintained a healthy weight for your body.

The only way to break the upward weight-gain cycle is to stop the dieting and deprivation and to learn a way of life that allows your body to lose fat (and the weight it represents). This requires a change of mind about what keeps you heavier than you want to be. As long as you believe that the only way to lose weight is to resist your appetite and go hungry, you are setting yourself up for defeat. Dieting sets up the cycle for binging and for lowering your metabolism so that you retain more fat from the calories you do eat. This leads you to the conclusion that you need to deprive yourself even more. These feelings of deprivation may set you up emotionally to rebel.

———————●———————

***Open your mind to changes
that will satisfy your appetite
without adding fat.***

If you have tried dieting and deprivation without lasting success at maintaining the healthy body weight you desire, why repeat patterns that don't work for you? Open your mind to making other kinds of changes that will satisfy your body's natural cravings for nourishment without adding excess fat.

Personal Evaluation

- Was there ever a time when you were able to maintain a healthy weight without excess fat on your body?
- When was the first time you dieted, restricting your eating so that your body's appetite was disregarded? After you began dieting did you reduce to a healthy weight, or did you begin a cycle of dieting and deprivation followed by a season of overeating and weight gain?
- How many different diets have you tried? Which ones satisfied you and kept your weight where you want it to be?
- Are you willing to open your mind to the possibility that dieting and deprivation contribute to maintaining excess weight?
- Are you willing to reeducate your mind and body to find a way to satisfy your body's cravings for nutritional satisfaction while losing fat?

Action

1. Today you will focus on getting an accurate record of your current eating habits. Remember, you are not focusing on what is "good" and "bad" in your eating habits. You are trying to get an accurate picture of what you ate today and your general eating habits during this season of life. Later you will

move into a new way of eating and use this evaluation for comparison, so it is to your advantage to be
as accurate as possible.

2. Title a sheet of paper "Eating Record." Across the
top of the page, set up columns with the following
headings: *When, What, Where, With Whom,* and
Why. Under *When* note the time you ate and how
long it took to eat. Under *What* note everything
you ate, including seasonings, spreads, and dressings. Under *Where* note where you were (location)
and anything you were doing simultaneously while
eating. Under *With Whom* note with whom you
ate. Under *Why* note whether you were physically
hungry and any other reason you had for eating at
that time. These reasons could range from "I didn't
want to leave any food on my plate because there
are children starving in Somalia" to "I passed the
chips and my hand just reached out before I
thought about it" to "I was bored and lonely, and
eating gave me some comfort." After you eat, without judging or condemning yourself, try to reflect
honestly on what factors are influencing you.

3. Think about four meals or treats you typically miss
most whenever you diet. This could be your favorite meal at your local fast-food restaurant, your
mother's Sunday supper, or a dessert you usually
find irresistible. Be sure you choose foods that have
been regular parts of your recent eating routines.

   Now you are going to make four coupons that
you can redeem at any time during these thirty
days for choosing to eat one of your familiar favorites. Use index cards to preplan departures from
the suggested eating adventures during this

thirty-day period. On each of the four cards, write out what you will allow yourself when you choose to depart from the ways of eating suggested during this adventure. For example, one coupon might read, "Go to Taco Bell for a Burrito Supreme, a taco, and a drink." Another might read, "Have a double-scoop ice cream cone." These are to be used whenever you want to go back to your old familiar ways of eating. However, limit yourself to the four coupons you create. If you use one, there is no need to condemn yourself and give up. Instead, go on with your preplanned program. Keep your coupons handy for later use.

Encouragement

By discovering the needs that eating meets in your life, you will be able to find healthy food alternatives that don't cause you to carry around excess fat.

Food for Thought

Enough is as good as a feast!
—Mary Poppins

DAY 4

Your Quest for a Less Fattening Lifestyle

Although you may think your goal is to lose ten pounds, this is not entirely true. Yes, losing ten pounds is the effect you desire. However, since you cannot directly "will away" ten pounds, your goal is to find a lifestyle that will result in weighing ten pounds less. Also, if you were to be precise, what you probably want to lose is ten pounds of excess body fat that is unattractive and unhealthy—not just ten pounds. Therefore, your adventure in losing just ten pounds could be viewed as a quest to find a less fattening lifestyle that you can live with.

There is a lot of talk these days about the merits of lowering the amount of fat you eat as a means of weight reduction. There are good reasons for this. A ground-breaking 1992 research study at Cornell University centered around a group who lowered their intake of fat, keeping the percentage of calories from fat under 25 percent of total calories eaten, while eating as much as they wanted. This group lost twice as much weight as a control group, who ate a relatively low-calorie diet. But their percentage of calories from fat was 35 percent to 40 percent of the total calories consumed.

———————•———————

You don't have to stop eating when you're still hungry.

———————————

The implications of this study can revolutionize the way you approach your lifestyle. If you accept these findings and adapt your approach to weight reduction, you may discover that you don't have to count calories and cut yourself off from food when you are really still hungry. Instead, you can eat good foods that are nutritionally sound to satisfy your physical hunger, as long as they are low in fat. This is the alternative to dieting and deprivation.

The first step toward developing a less fattening lifestyle is to become aware of how much fat there is in the foods you currently eat. Before you can make personal adjustments, you must have an accurate measurement of what you are accustomed to eating and what percentage of your total calories comes from fat.

Following are some simple ways you can begin to keep track of the percentage of fat in the calories you consume. There are handy pocket gauges available to calculate the fat-to-total-calories ratio. To use these, identify the number of calories per serving on the nutritional information label. Then locate the grams of fat per serving. Find these numbers on the gauge. (Two circles of card stock are attached together. The smaller, inner circle notes grams of fat, while the larger, outer circle notes calories.) When you line up grams to calories, the gauge will indicate percentage of calories from fat. These gauges can be found at many health-food stores or from health-care providers.

If you don't want to rely on using a gauge, here is a simple way you can calculate your fat-to-calorie ratio in your head. Each gram of fat equals nine calories. To calculate ratio of fat to calories, multiply the grams of fat by nine (giving you the number of calories from fat). Then divide the total number of calories by the number of calories from fat.

The nutritional information found on most packaging will look something like the following example. (This is a label from "light" mayonnaise.)

Serving Size . . . . 1 Tbsp.
Servings per Package 64
Calories 50
Protein 0
Carbohydrate 1g
Fat 5g
   Polyunsaturated 3g
   Saturated 1g

Cholesterol 0mg
Sodium 110mg

For this item you would note five grams of fat, multiplied by nine (calories per gram) = forty-five (calories per serving from fat). Since the total calories per serving amount to fifty, you have $^{45}/_{50}$ or $^{9}/_{10}$—90 percent of calories from fat.

If you don't carry a pocket calculator and aren't a whiz at computing figures in your head, try this trick. For the sake of ease and to give yourself a buffer in calculating fat intake, say that each gram of fat equals ten calories instead of the actual nine. Then it becomes easy to compute 2 grams of fat to twenty calories. Suppose the food you are checking has two grams of fat and 120 calories per serving. You know that 20 of the 120 calories come from fat. Since $^{20}/_{120} = ^{1}/_{6}$, about 16 percent of the calories come from fat. Remember, your goal is to keep your calories of fat/total calories ratio at or below $^{1}/_{4}$ or 25 percent.

Personal Evaluation

- Are you aware of what percentage of your total current calories comes from fat?
- Are you willing to familiarize yourself with nutritional information about what you are eating in order to reach your desired weight?
- Are you willing to monitor your percentage of fat in order to make changes that will help you lose weight?

Action

1. For the next twenty-four hours, keep track of the percentage of calories from fat in the foods you regularly eat. Be accurate about what you really eat, rather than adapting your figures toward what you think they should be. This time add a column for calories from fat/total calories ratio as follows: *When, What, Where, With Whom, Why, % Fat Calories.*
2. List every fast-food restaurant you frequent and what you usually order when you go there hungry. Use their nutritional information to calculate calories from fat. Most fast-food establishments have these readily available or will be happy to get you the information.

Encouragement

Becoming aware of the level of fat in your typical eating patterns will give you information you need. Now you can decide how you want to pare down to a less fattening lifestyle.

Food for Thought

You are what you eat!

Adopting a New
Pattern for Health

The pattern you follow in making anything in life will determine the form of what you create. Most Americans grew up with a nutritional pattern that looked something like figure 5.1.

Most of us were taught that as long as we had a good balance between these four food groups, we would be healthy. The pattern of the four basic food groups did not take into account the effect of a diet that was high in fat or the place of oils, fats, and sweets in the diet. The result was that many Americans who thought they were eating a healthy, balanced diet, according to this pattern, were actually eating a diet high in fat and refined sugars. We have

The Four Food Groups

Meat and Fish	Milk and Dairy Products
Grains, Breads, and Cereals	Fruits and Vegetables

Figure 5.1

since learned that this type of diet contributes to health problems (including excess weight).

On April 28, 1992 the U.S. Department of Agriculture released a new pattern of healthy nutritional guidelines. Instead of the old square, divided into four food groups, the new form is a triangle, divided into six food groups (see figure 5.2).

This new pattern represents a different way of thinking about what constitutes a healthy, balanced diet. It should result in a different way of life for those who seek to adapt their lifestyle to this new pattern for health.

If you are a typical American, you will probably notice that your diet consists of 35 percent to 40 percent fats, a dependence on red meat as your primary source of protein, and fewer whole grains, fruits, and vegetables than your body needs to maintain optimum health. Don't worry if this is the case. That will actually make losing ten pounds easier. If you eat a typically American high-fat diet, you have plenty of choices that will help you fulfill your nutritional needs,

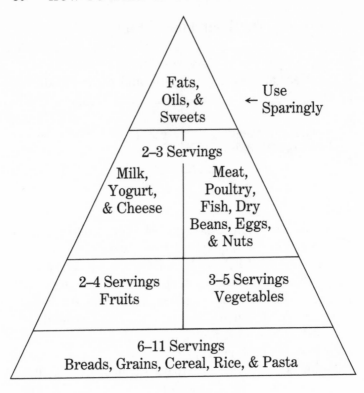

Figure 5.2

satisfy your hunger, and trim the fat from your diet and your body.

Personal Evaluation

- Can you remember being taught the four basic food groups as a pattern for healthy living?
- Do you recognize that using this pattern as a basis

for your understanding of a healthy diet has had an effect on the way you eat and think about food?

- Can you think of times when you justified eating things you felt were probably not a healthy choice by referring back to the four basic food groups pattern in your mind?
- If you were to adopt the new nutritional guidelines found in the pattern of the triangle, can you see how this would influence the way you think about food?
- How do you think your eating patterns would need to change to follow the nutritional guidelines found in the new pattern of the triangle?

Action

1. Study the nutritional guidelines found in the triangle until you can repeat the food groups and suggested daily servings from memory.
2. Look back at your eating records from days 3–5.
3. Analyze what you ate in terms of the pattern of the four basic food groups; that is, identify if you ate foods from those four groups and approximately how much.
4. Now analyze what you ate in terms of how it falls into the pattern set forth in the new triangle. Note how many servings and what percentage of your calories came from fats, oils, and refined sweets.

Encouragement

Realizing to what degree your eating patterns follow the old nutritional guidelines will help you identify where you need to make changes to lose excess fat.

Food for Thought

All changes, even the most longed for, have their melancholy; for what we leave behind us is a part of ourselves; we must die to one life before we can enter into another.

—Anatole France

6

Commit Yourself to the Adventure

By now you may be thinking, "OK, so when do I begin losing ten pounds?" You don't want to just think about losing weight; you want to do it! Today you begin translating what you have been learning into actions that affect your weight. But before taking action, you need to make a commitment to the adventure of discovering how to change your lifestyle. Following are the elements of this plan to which you are asked to commit yourself.

1. Your goal is to discover new ways of eating, being active, relating to food, planning your life, and visualizing yourself—all of which will help you lose excess fat.

2. Your goal is not to adhere to some prescribed "ideal" diet plan. Rather, you are becoming familiar with your current lifestyle as it affects your weight and looking for changes you can make to move your weight toward where you want it to be.

3. During the various phases of these thirty days, you will be focusing your attention on specific healthy food groups. The goal is to discover good foods to include in your eating routines to replace or reduce your dependence on fattening foods. As you move through the plan, you will add food groups. At the end of the thirty-day period, you will have one week of eating that follows a new pattern containing all food groups in healthy proportions.

4. During each phase you will be trying to discover new foods, new ways to prepare foods, or new ways of eating out. These will be less fattening than your past routine but should still satisfy you.

———————•———————

Focus on the goodness of new foods you are discovering.

5. Focus your attention on the goodness of the foods you are discovering or rediscovering, instead of thinking in terms of what you "can't" have. Appropriately, while you are moving through the remainder of the thirty days you are to eliminate foods prepared with refined sugar, other highly concen-

trated and high-calorie sweets, fats and oils such as
butter, and so on.
6. This program is an eating experience designed to
help you educate yourself and make personal
choices. These choices will lead to the creation of a
personalized lifestyle plan to keep you at a lighter
and healthier weight. No one can tell you what
your final lifestyle plan will look like. If you are
sharing this experience with a friend, the plans
each of you devise will be unique. However, each
plan will have these common elements:

- Realizing how your current lifestyle contributes
  to keeping you overweight
- Making choices to move in the direction of more
  nutritious, less fattening eating routines
- Developing a more active lifestyle
- Devising new strategies for dealing with emotional needs in ways other than finding sensual
  pleasure in eating
- Revising your schedule to allow yourself time
  to do the things that help you weigh less

Remember, the way to achieve the effect of weighing less is to learn to live differently. Since this is a
progressive program of discovery, your commitment
needs to be strong and deliberate so that you will
complete all thirty days. This is not a diet that you
will go back "on" if you "fall off." This truly is an
adventure in finding a satisfying way for you to live in
a body that carries around at least ten pounds less fat

than it does now. (Besides, you have your four coupons to use as needed.)

Your commitment to the lifestyle changes is what will result in the loss of weight. Therefore, you are encouraged to weigh yourself one last time today and then put away your scales until the end of the thirty-day period. If your commitment to completing this adventure in self-discovery is firm, you will do so. Weighing yourself along the way may be distracting or discouraging.

Personal Evaluation

- Are you willing to commit yourself to the adventure of discovering a less fattening way of life?
- Are you willing to put away your scale for thirty days and fully participate in this adventure, having faith that finding a less fattening lifestyle will result in weighing less?

Action

My Personal Commitment

I, _____ , am serious about my desire to lose weight and develop a less fattening lifestyle.

I am willing to invest at least thirty minutes a day, for each of the next thirty days, to focus on this transformation. I will plan to take this time every day (circle one): morning, lunchtime, afternoon, evening, or before bedtime. In addition, I am willing to reschedule my plans during this period to accommodate the kinds of activities that contribute to losing weight.

I understand that in order to reach this goal, I must be willing to grow on a personal level, to exercise the courage to look at myself honestly, and to endeavor to meet any challenges. I will do *my* best in all of these areas.

Since my goal is to lose just ten pounds, not to fit into some "perfect" mold, I will not focus my attention on how far I fall short of being the "ideal dieter" or having an ideal body. I will focus my attention on *moving forward* from where I am today, toward a lifestyle that keeps me weighing ten pounds less.

I make this commitment to myself this ___ day of _____ , 19___ .

_____
Signature

Encouragement

When you choose to commit yourself to the process that leads to weighing less, you are sure to end up weighing less—even if you don't watch your weight on the scales every day.

Food for Thought

One person with a commitment is worth a hundred with just an interest.

—Mary Crowley

Give Yourself Time
to Change

All true change takes the application of conscious effort practiced over time. Try to remember the last time you learned something new. It took a while for you to practice the new routine until it became a natural part of your life. You probably had to exert tremendous amounts of concentration to go through the paces. Once you became familiar with what you were learning, the process became something you did without conscious thought.

You will only be able to make lasting lifestyle changes by giving yourself time to learn new information, to practice new ways of living, and to think through the implications of the choices you are making.

Here are the areas in which you will need to give yourself time (in addition to the time spent reading each day's plan):

Grocery Shopping

Even if you are not used to doing your own grocery shopping, you will be exploring your food options by shopping as you move through your adventure. This necessitates doing your own food shopping or going along with the person who routinely does your shopping. Plan at least one hour for food shopping on days 8, 14, 19, and 24.

Preparation Time After Shopping

Plan an extra thirty minutes to one hour available for food preparation after shopping. When you come home from the grocery, you will be transforming much of your food into convenient form so that you will find it within easy reach when you need it. You will not be using many convenience foods and may be preparing foods in ways that are unfamiliar to you.

Cooking

This plan involves trying new foods and eating foods prepared in new ways. Therefore, you will probably need extra time to become familiar with food-preparation skills unfamiliar to you. Even if someone else cooks your food, your self-education would be incomplete if you didn't learn about low-fat cooking to determine the kinds of food and cooking methods you like or don't like.

Research

You probably eat out from time to time. When you plan to eat out, you will need to take time to discover menu alternatives available from your favorite restaurants or to locate new restaurants that offer the kinds of foods you are exploring. When you plan to try a new food, you may want to find a restaurant that prepares the food tastily. This way you will have some standard for appreciating how good the food can taste. Then you will not rule out a delicious food just because you didn't know how to prepare it properly.

Education

Part of your commitment is to learn new information about nutrition, exercise, and weight loss. You will need to take time to read, to visit the library or bookstore, to attend classes of interest to you (related to cooking or health), and to discuss what you are learning about your health with your support person.

Recess

One change in your life that you will make is to become more active on a daily basis. Just as children take breaks from sitting all day to get outside and move around, you will be scheduling two or three "recess" breaks into your daily routine. These are fifteen-minute breaks that you will use to get moving, hopefully in an enjoyable way.

Exercise

In addition to your daily recess breaks, schedule yourself set times of at least thirty minutes, three times per week (after day 21), for participating in a physical activity you enjoy.

Personal Evaluation

Are you willing to rearrange your schedule so that you can give yourself time to change and learn new ways of living?

Action

1. Sketch out a diagram that depicts twenty-four hours for each day in the remainder of your plan. If you already keep a calendar, refer to the plans you have recorded.
2. Fill in the hours that you regularly spend sleeping, eating, grooming, and taking care of other physical necessities.
3. Fill in the hours already committed to ongoing activities that you are not in a position to change, such as school, work, church, and so on.
4. Fill in all of the appointments you have planned for the next two weeks, such as going to the dentist or attending meetings, sporting events, and social events.

   Anything left open on your calendar should represent areas of opportunity. You can use these opportunities to focus your attention and energies on developing a new lifestyle that will leave you healthier and ten pounds lighter.
5. Make a list of the things that you need to do and/or want to do during this adventure.

6. Read over the list and rank each item with a $V = $ *very important* to me, $M = $ *moderately important* to me, or $O = $ *optional* (not really important to me).

7. Rearrange your schedule and make appointments to give yourself the time you will need to accommodate the following: grocery shopping = one hour or more, four times (days 8, 14, 19, and 24); preparation time after shopping = thirty minutes or more, four times; daily cooking and food preparation = an extra hour or more per day; researching restaurants = one to three hours total; education = thirty minutes to one hour a day, plus additional time for classes and so on as you like; recess = fifteen minutes, two or three times per day; exercise = thirty minutes to one hour, three times per week.

Encouragement

By making wise allowances of time, you are preparing to succeed in adopting a lifestyle that will keep you ten pounds lighter.

Food for Thought

Establishing priorities and using your time well aren't things you can pick up at Harvard Business School. If you want to make good use of your time, you've got to know what's important. Then give it all you've got.

—Lee Iaccoca

To begin the process of transforming the way you eat
and relate to food, you will spend days 8 through 13
eating primarily fruits and vegetables. If you have a
health condition that makes this inadvisable for you
(such as hypoglycemia or diabetes), consult your doctor or include whole grains. But continue to focus
your attention on developing your taste and apprecia-
tion for fruits and vegetables. Remember, U.S. Department of Agriculture guidelines recommend two to
four servings of fruit and three to five servings of
vegetables daily.

The purpose of this partial fast is not dietary. The
purpose is to help you break your dependence on the
wide range of foods you may eat that contribute to

your being overweight. This kind of partial fast is often used when people are trying to identify food allergies. Their diet is restricted; then foods are added one by one until the offending foods are identified. You will be following the same kind of process for yourself. You will start with a simple, natural diet of fruits and vegetables, then gradually add in other nutritious foods. However, you will not be looking for foods you are allergic to; you will be looking for good foods you may have neglected in favor of other fattening foods. Later, when you are designing your personalized plan, you can choose to substitute some of these new foods you enjoy for old ones that contribute to your weight problem.

———————•———————

Choose good foods you've neglected for fattening foods.

———————

Following are some of the benefits you will enjoy during your days of eating primarily fruits and vegetables.

1. You will have a reason to break from your routine. Most American diets are high in fat, processed foods, and refined sugar. You may be someone who sees meat as the centerpiece to every meal. When you see that you won't starve by eating a vegetarian diet for a few days, you will diminish your reliance on meat at every meal. By the end of the

thirty-day period, when you reincorporate meat into your meals, you will be more ready to enjoy smaller portions served with grains and vegetables.

2. You will discover delicious vegetarian main dishes that you can integrate into your meal plans.

3. You will probably lose water weight quickly and feel lighter. Although this weight loss is less important to your overall success than developing a taste for fruit and vegetables, you will be encouraged by feeling lighter.

4. You can use any sensation of hunger as an occasion to explore new vegetables and fruits. That way you will discover which ones satisfy you. You'll be amazed at your own creativity in coming up with vegetarian dishes, soups, and salads that you enjoy.

Personal Evaluation

- Are you willing to spend the next few days eating primarily fruits and vegetables?
- Do you have any kind of health problem that would make this kind of partial fast inadvisable?
- Are you willing to treat this as an adventure in finding fruits and vegetables to add to your menus?
- What vegetables do you like? (Make a list.)
- What fruits do you enjoy? (Make a list.)
- What vegetarian meals, soups, or entrées can you think of that you have tried and enjoyed?

Action

1. List all the fruits and vegetables you currently know you like. Make it your goal to add at least three new fruits and three new vegetables to this list. (The fruit could be presented in a new way, such as pineapple packed in its own juice rather than in syrup.)

2. Today you will shop for enough fruits and vegetables to keep yourself well fed until day 13. Allow yourself to eat any fruit or vegetable (including legumes) in its natural form. (That means without being processed with additional ingredients or added sugar.) You may want to consult the vegetable section of a cookbook you have on hand or access a vegetarian cookbook to help you plan what to buy. On a typical diet, you would have been advised to plan your meals before going to the market. However, since there are no restrictions on the kinds of fruits and vegetables you can eat in this plan, use this time to explore all the possibilities.

3. Start your shopping adventure with a positive attitude. Don't tell yourself about all the things you don't get to eat. (And certainly don't go down the aisles that have other foods.) Instead, look with new eyes on the abundance of fruits and vegetables available to us. Remind yourself of all the hungry people around the world who would be overjoyed to have access to this plenteous selection of fruits and vegetables.

———•———

Look with new eyes on the abundance of fruits and vegetables we have.

4. Shop in the produce section first. Buy at least three vegetables and one fruit that you have not tasted before. If there is a produce manager available, ask for suggested serving or cooking instructions. Choose vegetables you can eat raw, cooked, in salads, or in soups. Buy whatever you want. (You will be saving so much money usually spent on meat and convenience items that you can afford to splurge here.)

5. Move to the frozen food aisle, concentrating your attention on frozen fruits and vegetables. Beware of the ice cream and dessert cases! Take the time to explore the wide selection of vegetable dishes. If one has a mild sauce that is low in fat, try it. Remember, your purpose is to discover vegetables you will want to eat.

6. In the canned food section, be sure that the fruits you buy are canned only in water or in their own juices. Check out juices such as tomato and vegetable, which can be used as a starter for quick soups when you add fresh and frozen vegetables and seasonings. Don't forget to visit the international aisle for salsa, vegetables used in Chinese and Japanese dishes, and other items you might overlook.

7. If your market has a salad bar, you may want to make up an elaborate vegetable salad to help you

envision a nice meal from fresh fruits and vegetables. This brings up the question of sauces and dressings. For the sake of getting the most out of this exercise, you want to stay as simple as possible and remain fat free. You can use balsamic vinegar, lemon juice, and other natural seasonings; or you may want to use a small amount of fat-free salad dressing. Plan to use salsa or other seasoned vegetables to top baked potatoes instead of high-fat alternatives.

8. When you come home, immediately prepare your vegetables for handy snacks. Cut up fresh vegetables such as carrots, bell peppers, celery, tomatoes, cucumbers, and so on for times when you want to munch. Store these in a handy dish or sealed plastic bags.

Encouragement

By filling your shopping cart, refrigerator, freezer, and cupboards with wholesome foods today, you are helping yourself make good food choices tomorrow.

9

Health in Motion

If you have a sedentary lifestyle, this factor probably contributes as much to your carrying excess body fat as the way you eat. Poor eating habits and lack of physical activity seem to go together. When you over-eat or eat foods high in fat and refined sugars, you feel sluggish. If you are overweight, you may be physically uncomfortable carrying around your extra weight or embarrassed to be seen by others. Therefore, you may be unmotivated to get moving initially. The more you neglect physical activity, the less likely you are to feel a natural desire to get moving. Therefore, you must convince your mind to get your body moving.

Once you make an intellectual decision to increase

your physical activity level, you will need to practice the habit of moving more, initially as an act of your will. However, it doesn't take long before the cycle begins working in your favor. Your body will start feeling the good effects of moving around more. You will find that you have more energy, generally feel better, and are less tense.

Once you begin to enjoy the benefits of increased activity, you may realize that you can use exercise to relieve tension instead of immediately putting something in your mouth. Your initial decision to increase your activity level prepares you to later choose an exercise program you may have been hesitant to try.

———————•———————

Use exercise to relieve tension rather than eating.

———————————

Today's focus is not on starting an aggressive exercise program. Most health-care professionals agree that a good program for staying physically fit includes twenty- to thirty-minute sessions of aerobic exercise three or four times per week. This may be the standard plan for health, but you are focusing on starting where you are and making changes that will improve your health and help you lose weight. Therefore, don't worry about the "standard" exercise program for now. Instead, focus on evaluating your current activity level and increasing your activity level a little bit every day.

Following are some of the many facts you can use to motivate yourself to get moving a bit more than you are used to.

1. The combination of eating healthfully and becoming more physically active is far more effective in losing fat and improving physical fitness than just dieting.
2. Physical activity relieves physical and emotional tension, often helping to alleviate stress-related symptoms (such as headaches) as well. Bottled emotions, anxiety, stress, and tension contribute to all kinds of physical and emotional disorders and diseases. Regular exercise can prevent or relieve many related health problems.
3. Many people react to stress by eating rather than moving. If you routinely eat when stressed or tense, you could be pounds lighter just by choosing to do something physical before you resort to eating. Chances are good that the exercise will reduce stress. Then you can avoid many occasions of stress-related eating and thus lose weight.
4. Exercise has been proven to elevate moods and often helps to alleviate some forms of depression.

Personal Evaluation

- Turn back in your notebook to the activity record you made on day 2. You should have tracked your physical movements enough to have a record of your typical activity level for a normal workday and a day off. If you have the records, review your movements.

- Recall a time when you were more physically active. What kinds of movement or routines increased your activity level then?
- Have you fallen into the cycle of allowing a lack of physical exercise to keep you from feeling like moving? Or are you embarrassed at the thought of being more physically active?

Action

1. Look at your daily paths of movement (where you go to and from each day). Plan to increase your activity level in little ways along your normal path. Some suggestions would include parking farther from your destination, taking the stairs instead of the elevator, answering the telephone farthest from you in your home instead of a portable phone or the nearest extension, walking children to and from school on days when weather permits instead of driving them, and so on.
2. Plan to take tiny activity breaks whenever you are sitting for long periods of time. If you spend hours in front of the television, use the commercial breaks to jump rope, stretch, walk around the house, jog in place, or engage in other active movement. If you travel long distances by car, take planned breaks to walk and stretch. Choose one activity to do during sitting time, and commit yourself to incorporating this activity into your life.
3. Play with your family and friends in a physical

manner. Plan one time each week that you can play together physically. This doesn't mean you have to do an exercise program together. Rather, think of fun activities your family enjoys that are physically active. Some suggestions would include dancing, bowling, roller-skating, walking on the beach, taking nature hikes, wrestling with small children, having fun on the playground, playing catch with a ball, trying croquet, swimming, and so on.

———————•———————

When the bell rings, take a recess!

4. Make the decision to take two or three fifteen-minute recesses per day. You remember recess. You were working hard at school; then the bell would ring and everyone would go outside to play and run for a few minutes. Use a bell or set a timer to announce recess (preplan the times according to your schedule and job demands). Then, when the bell rings, head outside; or at least walk away from your desk and get moving.

   Don't fall for the self-delusion that you don't have time for recess. The truth is that by taking a physical break of this type, you will be more productive in whatever you do during the rest of the day.

5. Schedule your recess times now and write them in your calendar. Get yourself a timer or an alarm to alert you to recess times, and use it for the remain-

der of the thirty days. Once this becomes a routine part of your life, you may not need a bell. But for now it will prove helpful.

6. Make another chart like the one you used on day 2, which tracks your physical activity during the course of one twenty-four-hour period. Tomorrow follow yourself through the day, including the activities you noted today, and monitor your new level of activity. The columns you will use are the same as before: *When, What Motion, Where, Why, Emotional Feelings*, and *Physical Feelings*.

Encouragement

By making the intellectual and deliberate choice to enhance your health by increased physical activity, you are paving the way to enjoying exercise. Then you can reap the many benefits a regular exercise program provides.

Food for Thought

Take short steps. A lot of people fail because they try to take too big a step too quickly.

—Zig Ziglar

DAY
10

No Need to Rebel

One of the dangers of dieting is the rebellion trap. This human flaw was demonstrated way back in the beginning when the first restrictive diet was announced. God said to Adam and Eve, "You can eat anything in the garden, except the fruit on the tree in the center of the garden. Of that tree you shall not eat, or you will surely die." Well, you know the rest of the story. What one food item became absolutely irresistible? Did they focus on the wide range of good foods available in abundance? Nope! They headed for the one food they were told *not* to eat—even though they had it on good authority that eating it would kill them. (Does this sound a bit too familiar?)

Well, you probably know from personal experience

that human nature hasn't changed from that day to this. Just let someone give you a list of foods you cannot eat, and suddenly that forbidden fruit will become the object of desire.

———————•———————

***You will encounter no lists of
forbidden foods in this
adventure.***

During this thirty-day period you will find no reason to rebel. You will notice that there are no lists of forbidden foods (which may encompass the source of much of your pleasure in life!). Rather, you are directed to focus your attention on many of the good foods you may be missing. Since, in order to succeed in losing weight, we need to take human nature into account, you were instructed on day 2 to create four coupons. These coupons contain notes about your favorite foods—those you have missed the most when you dieted in the past. These coupons are for you to redeem whenever you choose during the thirty days. If you are feeling deprived or are distracted by missing your familiar foods, use one of your coupons to entitle you to have that meal or food.

Don't fall into the trap of seeing the use of these coupons as cheating. You are not on a diet. You are experimenting with good foods to help you make future choices about healthy foods you can enjoy. Then it will be easier to let go of some of your familiar, more fattening foods. Even by using your food coupons during these thirty days, you are still eating better than you were when you relied on these foods more often. Also, you will not trigger guilt-related binging, which can happen when you diet and then have a food you rely on for pleasure. It's OK; having a favorite food four times during this period will not defeat your purposes in devising a new, less fattening lifestyle.

You are in charge of discovering some satisfying but less fattening foods, activities, and ways of life. At the end of this program you will look at the eating and activity records you kept at the beginning. You will use the knowledge and experience you have gained to help you decide what changes you can make to retain your new weight.

Remember, this is a guided transition program, not a diet. You can use these exercises to whatever degree you choose to help you identify new foods, new ways of eating and cooking, new activities, and new ways of thinking about yourself. The goal is to use this time to reevaluate your eating habits, lifestyle, and activities to devise a satisfying life. Since no one is forcing you, there's no need to rebel.

Personal Evaluation

- How much of a role did rebellion play in thwarting your previous attempts to lose weight?
- How does designing your own program and using this as an eating adventure help defuse the rebellion you usually battle?

- Are you able to adjust your thinking to focus on all the good things you are discovering you may like and can have, or are you still focused primarily on what you cannot have?

Action

Think about your coupons. Remind yourself that you can use them whenever you choose. If you want to plan when to redeem them, go ahead and schedule those times. If you want to keep them to use whenever you desire, put them in a place where you will carry them with you. Once you redeem a coupon, mark it so that you know it is used.

Encouragement

Don't panic! No one is trying to take away your favorite foods forever. Knowing that you have control over choosing when to eat your familiar (although possibly fattening) favorites will help you discover the freedom to sometimes choose healthier alternatives.

Food for Thought

The important thing is this: to be able at any moment to sacrifice what we are for what we could become.

—Charles du Bois

DAY
11

Learning to Listen to Your Body

Eating is often done compulsively and impulsively. We respond to many internal and external stimuli other than hunger. Learning to listen to the hunger signals given by your body and to eat in response to hunger may revolutionize your relationship to food.

Hunger is a physical sensation rather than an emotional response or a reaction to a sensual or social stimulus. In our society, eating is often used to feed emotional hungers for love and comfort. It is also a social pastime. If you learn to recognize when you are eating for emotional or social reasons, you can give yourself the choice of fulfilling your emotional and social needs in other ways that don't cause you to be overweight.

"Unconscious" eating puts on extra pounds. It is not related to addressing legitimate hunger. To become aware of your unconscious eating, make a practice of taking your food to a designated place and sitting down while you eat. When you first begin to do this, you may be surprised to discover how many times your hands lift food to your mouth without conscious thought.

Many people in our culture never allow themselves to experience physical hunger because they routinely eat before their body becomes hungry. Others constantly feel hungry, never able to satisfy their appetites even though they may eat constantly. This may be due to undernourishment from the things they are overeating. When your body is in a constant state of craving, but you continue to feed yourself things that do not satisfy the nutritional needs of your body, your hunger signals do not serve you as they were intended.

Part of the reasoning behind eating primarily fruits and vegetables during the first phase of your program is to give you the opportunity to feel hunger signals. By learning to recognize hunger signals, you will be in a position to make eating choices that are more in tune with your body. You don't want to go hungry as you have in the past when you dieted. Instead, you want to listen to the physical hunger signals given by your body and to satisfy your hunger at that time. Also, by eating nutritious fruits and vegetables, you will break the cycle of dependence on processed foods that please your tastebuds and fill your stomach, but don't satisfy real nutritional needs.

———————●———————

You can eat as much as you want.

You will not starve. If you have gone through seasons of deprivation, your mind may associate hunger with painful emotional memories and therefore cause you to avoid hunger at all costs. You must change your mind about hunger to benefit your life today. Try to see hunger as your friend. If you learn to listen to your hunger and eat in response to hunger signals, you will lose weight.

Sometimes when you feel that you want something, you may be thirsty rather than hungry. When you get a physical sensation that you think is hunger, try having a drink of water or juice.

Personal Evaluation

- How can you recognize when you eat for emotional or social reasons rather than to satisfy physical hunger?
- When is the last time (if ever) you recall feeling the physical sensation of hunger?
- Do you constantly feel hungry for something, even if you eat continually?
- Do past experiences of hunger or deprivation give you a strong aversion to allowing yourself to ever feel hungry?

- Are you willing to try to see hunger as a resource, helpful for guiding you to a healthy way of eating?

Action

1. Look back at your eating records, where you noted what you ate and why. Circle every time you ate because you were hungry. Remember, the point is to learn to respond to your body and eat whenever you are hungry. When you do feel hungry, eat until your hunger is comfortably satisfied.
2. For the remainder of the thirty days, try to catch yourself before indulging in unconscious eating. If you still want to eat that morsel that seemed to leap into your hand, take it to your eating place and eat it sitting down.
3. Across the top of a sheet of paper write these words: *Emotional Hunger, Physical Hunger,* and *Social Stimulus.* After each time you eat (while you are still sitting down), jot down what you ate under the column that represents what you believe to be the reason you ate at that time. If your reasons were social or emotional, specify what prompted you to eat at the time. An example of emotional hunger might be: Used coupon for hot fudge sundae because I was upset after argument with Mom. An example of a social stimulus might be: Visited Judy; she offered me lunch and I didn't want to hurt her feelings.

———————————•———————————

Eat until your appetite is satisfied and hunger abates.

———————————

4. Begin to practice listening to your body's hunger signals to decide when to stop eating. As you eat, become aware of when your body feels satisfied and hunger abates. If you eat more slowly, you may be able to notice this point before overeating.
5. Try to move toward waiting until you are hungry to eat. See if you can increase the times you eat in response to hunger and decrease the times you eat in reaction to emotions or social stimulus. Keep recording why you are eating for a few days until you become aware of listening to your body's hunger signals.
6. There will be times when you are not sure whether you are hungry or not. When you aren't sure, try waiting twenty minutes or drinking a glass of water. Then see if the feeling is truly a hunger signal.

Encouragement

Once you learn to listen to your body and respond to true hunger signals, you will find losing weight easier.

DAY

12

Good Sensations

Your body has five senses: touch, sight, hearing, smell, and taste. Many people who overeat tend to get the majority of their sensations of pleasure from taste and relatively little pleasure from their remaining senses. If all the pleasure seems to have gone out of your life because you are not currently eating indiscriminately, you have not been getting enough pleasure from your other senses.

———————•———————

Find pleasure from all five of your senses.

Touch

If you are overweight, you may deprive yourself of the pleasure of touching and being touched by others because you are ashamed of your body. Whatever your weight, you need and deserve to be touched. If you cannot bring yourself to allow others to touch you, here are some ideas of how you can give yourself the gift of touch.

1. Take a bubble bath.
2. After the bath, dry yourself with a thick, fluffy towel. (Perhaps buy one especially for you.)
3. Dust yourself with bath powder, or use other after-bath products.
4. Soak your feet in a foot massager.
5. Generously rub lotion on hands, feet, face, and body.
6. Give yourself a facial.

Following are some ideas that involve touching and being touched by others.

1. Give and receive hugs.
2. Get a massage, facial, manicure, or pedicure.
3. Have your hair washed and styled at a salon.
4. Spend more time being intimate with your spouse.
5. Give or receive a backrub.

Sight

1. Read a great book. (This uses eyesight and imaginative sight.)
2. Visit an art museum.

3. Take a nature walk or go bird-watching.
4. Look at a child sleeping.
5. Go stargazing.
6. Watch clouds go by.
7. Watch waves crashing on the beach or a river winding by.

Hearing
1. Listen to your favorite music.
2. Call a friend with whom you've lost touch and enjoy hearing his or her familiar voice.
3. Listen to relaxation tapes that re-create beautiful sounds of nature, such as a rushing waterfall, sea sounds, a forest at night, and so on.
4. Reduce the noise around you and enjoy quiet sounds.

Smell
Your sense of smell may tend to lead you in the direction of food, and that is one of the blessings of life. However, there are many other ways to enjoy your sense of smell.

1. Wear perfume or cologne with a fragrance you enjoy.
2. Stop to smell the flowers. Roses, gardenias, lilacs—God has filled our world with wonderful and distinct fragrances. Take some time to appreciate particular flowers.
3. Simmer potpourri.
4. Burn candles with fragrance.

5. Clean out the musty odors around you (in home, office, and car). Then spray air freshener.

Personal Evaluation

- Use percentages to estimate how many of your sensual pleasures currently come from taste and eating and how many from each of your other four senses.
- Are you willing to try some new ways of experiencing pleasure to compensate for some of the taste sensations you are choosing to forego during this phase of your thirty-day period?

Action

1. For each of the senses of touch, sight, hearing, and smell, choose three things you will do each week to give you pleasure.
2. Do one pleasurable activity from each category today, and continue to focus on giving yourself good sensations other than taste when you are thinking of some tastes you may be missing.

Responding to What You're Missing Most

By now your adventure with fruits and vegetables may be losing some of its novelty. You are probably becoming aware of a desire for some of the foods you are missing. That is good! Identifying the foods you truly miss provides you with information you will use later to help you make good choices. It is also helpful to take note of those foods you don't particularly miss, even though you haven't been eating them.

At the end of this plan you will be choosing which fattening foods to eat less than you previously did, as well as which new foods to include in your regular eating patterns. You will also be looking for low-fat alternatives for high-fat foods. By taking note of what you miss most, you will know what foods you really are not willing to eliminate from your regular eating patterns. By taking note of some high-fat, processed foods full of empty calories or food products high in refined sugar that you don't miss, you will identify a way to cut fat from your diet (and in turn, your body) without feeling that you are missing out on something important to you.

Personal Evaluation

- What foods do you miss the most?
- What foods do you feel your body may be craving: grains, pasta, bread, red meat, poultry, fish, cereal?
- If you used one of your familiar foods coupons, did eating that food have the same taste and feel as it did before? How was it different?
- What foods do you find that you are not missing noticeably?
- Which, if any, of these foods you are not consciously missing are high in fat, highly processed, or high in refined sugar?
- Which restaurants do you miss going to, or which menu items do you miss from a particular restaurant?

Action

1. List all the foods you can think of that you used to eat at home on a regular basis.
2. List all the foods you can recall that you used to snack on regularly.

3. List all the menu items you used to enjoy at every restaurant you frequented.
4. Go through your lists and circle any items that have more than 30 percent of the total calories from fat.
5. Go through your lists and draw a box around any items that have refined sugar as a primary ingredient.
6. Now review all your lists. Rate each item on a scale of one to ten in terms of how important this food is to you. (A rating of one would mean that you wouldn't care if you never tasted it again; a rating of five would mean that you miss it but could live without it without feeling deprived. A rating of ten would mean that you miss it, you long for the day when you can taste it again, and you would miss it terribly if you never had it again.)
7. As you continue through these thirty days, keep this list and add foods to it as they come to mind. Then circle, box, and rate each one accordingly. You will use this evaluation to help you make healthy choices near the end of the program.

Encouragement

By becoming aware of those things that really matter to you, you can hold on to what is important, reduce the fattening things that don't matter much, and lose weight without feeling deprived.

Exploring the
Goodness of Grains

Today you will expand your eating repertoire to include grains, pasta, breads, cereals, and other grain products. For the next few days you will still eat whatever fruits and vegetables you like, in addition to grain products. Your focus over the next few days is to expand your familiarity with the wide range of satisfying options you have for healthful eating with this category of foods. You will be exploring and introducing yourself to new tastes, textures, and ways of cooking and thinking about grains. For this reason, try not to fall back into eating your old favorites. Instead, purposefully look for new items as you shop and eat out.

———————•———————

Grains are central to nutritious eating.

———————————

Grains are central to nutritious eating. Grains and grain-related products are recommended as the basis for a healthy diet. You should recall that the U.S. Department of Agriculture's triangle model recommends six to eleven servings of foods from the grain category as the basis for a healthy diet.

In our culture, grains are primarily thought of as a side dish. Your goal over the next few days is to change your mind about and your taste in grains, elevating them to the central place of importance to your daily eating patterns.

As you set out to shop for grains and grain products you may want to go to a health-food store, where you will find grains in bulk and packaged with seasoning. You may also have better access to a store employee who can educate you on various cooking methods and suggested seasonings.

Following are some grains you may want to try.

Rice

Try long-grain white converted rice, aromatic rice (such as Basmati or Texmati), short-grain brown rice, and wild rice. If you like, try the "instant" rice, both brown and white, as well as simple long-cooking rice you can buy in bulk.

Millet

Millet is a grain that has been cultivated for centuries. You may be more familiar with the uncooked small round grain as a component in birdseed. However, millet is delicious cooked and used any time you would think of using rice. Cooked millet is light and fluffy with a nutty flavor. It's great with vegetable stir-fry, even in soufflé.

Whole Wheat

Wheat berries ground into flour can also be enjoyed cooked whole or sprouted and used in salads. These are chewier than brown rice in texture and are great for giving body to soups and stews.

Cracked Wheat

Cracked wheat is whole wheat ground into a coarse texture. This can be a delicious, hearty breakfast cereal when cooked with chopped dates or raisins.

Bulgur

Bulgur consists of wheat berries that have been cooked, cracked into pieces, and then dried. Bulgur does not need to be cooked. It can be soaked in water or broth and used in cold salads as well as in soups.

Rye

Most people are familiar with the strong flavor of rye bread. Rye is often used in recipes from cookbooks featuring international cuisine. Of course, you can enjoy various intensities of rye breads and crackers.

Barley

Since barley in its whole state has a hard, outer shell, this is usually removed in a process called pearling. Pearled barley has lost some of the nutrients, but is no longer tough. Some barley found in health-food stores has not been as highly processed as commercial barley, thus may be slightly darker. Barley's chewy texture and mild flavor make it a welcome addition to soups and casseroles. Roasted barley flour also makes tasty bread and rolls.

Oats

Oat flakes and rolled oats are most often thought of as the basis for hot breakfast cereal or granola. All it takes to make a meal is to add cooked fruit and perhaps a bit of honey or sweetener. You can also use oat flour in breads and biscuits.

Corn

Corn is highly versatile and was used here as a staple long before the founding of this country. You can eat fresh corn on the cob, pop corn kernels (try an air popper or microwave oven), or use cornmeal as a breakfast porridge by boiling it in water. Cornbread and corn tortillas are popular fare. You could also form a cornmeal crust for main-dish casseroles.

Buckwheat

Buckwheat kernels have a rich, nutty flavor. Buckwheat's flavor complements winter vegetable stews containing root vegetables, sage, and marjoram. You can buy it plain or roasted in coarse, medium, or fine grinds.

Couscous

Couscous is really pellets of pasta. However, it is often found with other grains or in the international section of some markets.

Pastas

Since you are exploring new options, why not have some fun with pastas? Try new shapes, colors, and brands. Try whole wheat pasta, egg noodles, and fresh pastas found in the refrigerated case. You may even want to try making your own pastas. Also, try using pasta in new ways. For example, it can serve as the basis for cold salads without mayonnaise, served with vegetables and a pasta sauce.

If you have told yourself that you must stay away from pasta, try to rethink this. What you probably need to stay away from are the high-fat dressings, such as mayonnaise, which typically go with pasta salads and high-fat sauces or meats that may accompany other pasta dishes. Pasta can be great if you use it in new ways.

Breads

Try some new varieties of whole-grain breads. If you are a person who balks at the higher prices of whole-grain or fresh-baked breads, give yourself this luxury. You are not spending money on the meats you usually have. Later you may want to allow yourself higher-priced breads as you cut down on the amount of expensive processed foods and red meat you eat.

Boxed Grain Products

There are many boxed varieties of grain dishes available on the shelf of grocery stores and health-food stores. The Near East label carries several grain dishes available with the spices that make these grains favorites in international and Middle Eastern recipes. More traditional labels such as Rice-A-Roni have spiced grain dishes as well. Since getting the right spices will determine how well you enjoy various grains, you may find it helpful to begin tasting these. However, be aware of the ingredients. Avoid packages that have fats and dairy products added. Look for those with combinations of grains, pasta, and spices.

Cereals

Remember that you are adding grains, not refined sugars, at this time. You may want to explore the cereal aisle for whole-grain cereals to add to your daily fare (for instance, shredded wheat). However, most prepared cereals are high in added sugar and fats. You may want to look for cereals at a health-food store so that you are not distracted from your focus on wholesome grains.

Personal Evaluation

- Which of the aforementioned grains were a part of your regular eating patterns before starting this adventure?
- Have you thought of grains primarily as a side dish?
- Are you open to expanding the role you allow grains, breads, pastas, and cereals to play in your diet?

Action

1. Go shopping for fruits, vegetables, and grain products.
2. Plan meals that depend on these foods. You may want to get some new cookbooks that feature vegetarian recipes.
3. List every new grain product you try, how you cooked it, and how well you liked it.

Encouragement

By enriching your life with the goodness of grain, you will find your appetite satisfied. Also, you will be better able to conceive of reducing your dependence on high-fat foods and meats.

15

Planning to Weigh Less

Planning gives you great opportunities for making choices that will help you weigh less. Often you will indulge in fattening choices when you find yourself hungry at the wrong time and place. You can make eating and activity choices that protect you from situations you may find difficult to resist.

Following are some ways that planning can help you make lifestyle changes for weighing less.

Plan to Accommodate Routine "Fat Traps"

If you take time to reflect on the routines of your lifestyle, you will be able to identify certain places or activities where you tend to eat fattening food or to overeat. By predicting these events you will be in a better position to accommodate them.

For example, suppose you are planning to have dinner at your grandmother's home. Her meals are always irresistible, and you know her old heart will be broken if you don't have second helpings. You don't have to stop visiting Grandma, but you need to plan around that meal. You could plan to be especially conscious of eating low-fat foods for a few days prior to your visit.

Plan for Those High-Fat, High-Calorie, Low-Satisfaction Moments

One woman who works for a candy company was asked daily to "test" a sample from each batch of candy. She didn't have a desire for chocolate before it was put before her. However, she found that if she were hungry, she would always accept. She started bringing an apple and hard candies to work with her. Each day she now eats her apple immediately before the candy is brought around to the workers. If she still wants something sweet, she sucks on the hard candy (which takes longer and packs far fewer calories and fat). Once a week she plans to taste the candy and enjoys it when she does.

Another pertinent suggestion is to notice parts of your meals that don't do much to satisfy you, but that are very fattening. For example, if you are going to be eating at a Mexican restaurant, you could eat thousands of high-fat calories in chips and salsa while waiting to order. Instead, put a breath mint in your mouth. Breath mints and salsa taste awful together.

Plan to Eat Out

Take note of your plans to go out with friends for entertainment and any times you will be eating out. Prepare to suggest restaurants with menus containing items that you enjoy, but that aren't going to pile on fat and excess calories.

Anticipate Changes in Your Appetite

If you know you always get hungry mid-morning, plan to take a healthy snack with you. Otherwise, you may find the candy vending machine irresistible.

Many women find that their appetite fluctuates predictably with their menstrual cycle. If you happen to know which days each month you will be more hungry than usual, plan to stock up on healthy snacks. Be sure your supplies of fattening treats aren't in the house at that time.

Plan to Have Treats As a Matter of Choice

By learning to make your eating choices in advance, you spare yourself from eating that seems out of control and that may produce guilt. There will be times when you will still indulge in fattening treats as a matter of choice. Your aim is to do so less compulsively, perhaps less often, and without triggering a cycle of guilty binge eating. The best way is to plan your treats. If you are in the habit of having a special treat every night, you would be pounds lighter by choosing to plan your treat once or twice a week.

Plan for Shopping Trips

Plan your shopping list before going to the grocery store. Be sure you have enough food to keep from having to go shopping several times each week. The less often you are in the store, the less you will be persuaded by all the marketing campaigns to buy and eat foods that will make you gain excess weight.

Always plan to eat before grocery shopping. If your hunger is fully satisfied, you will find it easier to stick to your shopping list.

Make Eating Decisions in Advance

For the most part, you want to learn to make eating decisions in advance. Choose the kinds of foods that you will bring into your home. Choose what you want to eat before you go into the kitchen. If you are hungry or just want something to eat, decide what you want; then go get it. Sit down at your eating place and eat. Stop going into the kitchen hungry and rummaging around to see what strikes your fancy. When you do that, you are more inclined to eat impulsively.

Personal Evaluation

- Which of these planning strategies do you already employ?
- Are you willing to practice planning in ways that help you anticipate trouble spots?

- Are you willing to try these strategies to see which ones help you lose weight?

Action

1. Review your daily routine. Identify any times when you are particularly susceptible to overeating or eating impulsively. Devise your own plan to deal with the challenges you face daily. Write out your plan to deal with daily "fat traps."
2. Review your plans and appointments for the next month. Identify any times or events that have potential for being food-indulgent experiences. Highlight the previous days to cut back on fat and calories to compensate.
3. Plan your grocery shopping trips on your calendar. Take time to write out a list. Plan to eat before shopping.
4. Plan your treats. Consider your coupons, which you may plan to use for a special familiar meal or food during this period. Look ahead on your calendar for after the adventure is finished, and schedule treats less often than you routinely had them before you began these thirty days.
5. Make a list of your ideas for how to resist high-fat, high-calorie foods when they don't really matter to you.

Encouragement

Your willingness to plan ahead will make it easier for you to shed the ten pounds you want to lose.

DAY
16

Pantry and Menu Planning

If you practice writing out weekly menus and shopping from your menu, you will save money at the market and help yourself lose weight. You don't have to slavishly obey your menu plan. You can adapt your meals or switch around their order. Menu planning can help you to be less inclined to head for the fast-food place. Also, planning your meals helps to keep you satisfied with good foods so that you eat impulsively much less often. Menu planning is especially helpful when you are familiarizing yourself with new foods. This adventure will be more fun if you enjoy looking for good recipes and anticipating trying new ways of cooking and eating.

———————————•———————————

Anticipate new ways of cooking and eating.

—————————————————

Menu planning is not just for the cook in the family. It is your chance to decide what you want to eat, whether you will be eating at home or at a restaurant, and whether you will rely on home cooking or prepared meals (frozen dinners and so on).

Following are ideas that will help you plan simple menus.

1. Make a list of meals you cook or eat on a regular basis. Think in terms of listing main dishes with meat, casseroles, and vegetarian dishes, along with foods you like to have with that particular meal.
2. Look at your schedule and the schedule of others in your household for the upcoming week.
3. Note which meals will be eaten at home, with ample preparation time; which meals will have to be rushed because of other commitments; when you plan to eat out; and other influences on the time you have for preparation and eating.
4. Select meals from your list of favorites, including quick, simple meals for days when time is limited. Perhaps you will choose frozen meals or even fast food for some nights. (Remember, you do have a choice about what you order, even in fast food.) List staples for breakfasts and lunches as well as planning for healthy snacks each day.

5. Write your menu plan ahead for one or two weeks. Post this somewhere in your kitchen. You may find it helpful to use an erasable calendar with dry erase markers. These can be affixed to the refrigerator with magnets and will allow you to amend your menu plans as schedules change.

6. From your menu, write a complete list of items you will need from the store. This becomes your shopping list, to which you add any items from your pantry that have been used up in the previous week.

7. For help in planning your pantry and menus, I suggest reading *The Monday to Friday Cookbook* by Michele Urvater (New York: Workman Publishing, 1991). Ms. Urvater is a corporate professional cook whose recipes are all low in fat and cholesterol but high in flavor. She also teaches planning methods that will help you learn to change your eating, shopping, and cooking habits.

Personal Evaluation

Are you willing to practice planning menus for a while to help you focus on eating healthy new meals, instead of just reverting to the old, familiar foods that contributed to your being overweight?

Action

1. Since you just went shopping two days ago, you don't need to go again. Go through this menu-planning process in preparation for the next time you

go shopping (day 19). You can plan to include dairy products that are fat free or low fat in your menus, since you will be adding these at that time.

2. Go through the menu-planning process completely, including your old favorite family meals on your initial list of meals. Later you will adapt your favorite foods list to your advantage.

   You should end up with the following:

   - A written list of favorite familiar meals
   - A schedule of the upcoming time period, highlighted with notes of the kind of meal you have time for each day
   - A list of breakfasts and lunches you plan to have
   - A posted menu of meals and snacks for the coming week
   - A shopping list of ingredients needed for menu planning

Encouragement

If you will practice learning to plan your menus, you will have greater control over what you eat and the effect your meals have on your body.

17

Creating a Less Fattening Kitchen

How you cook as well as what you cook may be contributing to your excess weight. There are ways to redesign the use of your kitchen and revise what you keep on hand, helping you lose weight and keep it off.

Pantry

Your pantry consists of what you have on hand from which the regular, basic staples of your diet are taken. If your pantry items include gourmet cookies, potato chips, and other high-fat, high-calorie items, you will predispose yourself to having to fight off temptation every time you open a cupboard or look in the refrigerator. *Redesign your pantry* to rely on highly nutritious, low-fat foods that will make up the basis of your new eating patterns. This is not to say that you will never bring certain foods into your home just because they are fattening. You may choose to do that occasionally, but these kinds of items are being removed from the category of everyday items in your pantry.

Cookware

The following items will help you cook in ways that don't add extra fat in the cooking process:

A *vegetable steamer* will allow you to enjoy cooked vegetables with no added fat. Some steamers are complete units, having a cooking bowl and timer. The more common type is the insert you place on the bottom of a saucepan to hold the vegetables above boiling water.

A *nonstick skillet* will allow you to cook without having to fry foods in oil. The nonstick surface also makes cleanup easier.

Storage Containers

If you have storage containers that make good foods easy to keep on hand (such as a *fresh-vegetable tray*), you will be more inclined to prepare healthy snacks. Having a *sealable salad bowl* will encourage you to keep salad available.

Food Preparation Helps

If your new choices of food are not easy to prepare, chances are that you will revert to the old ways of eating that contributed to your being overweight.

Following are some items that make food preparation easier.

A *salad spinner* is used to dry lettuce leaves after washing. You can wash salad greens in bulk, dry them, and prepare a basic salad for use over the course of several days if the greens are stored properly.

If you find that you enjoy sprouted beans and grains, you may want to sprout your own (mung beans, lentils, radish, wheat, alfalfa, and so on). *Sprouters* are easy to use and available at most health-food stores. This is a fun project for youngsters who may be curious about your new adventures in eating.

Food processors are helpful; but if you find you don't use your food processor because it takes too much effort to clean and put away, try an alternative. There are mini food processors or mini choppers. Some are used to grind coffee beans and can be used to chop nuts, herbs, and other small items. There is also the kind of hand-held model that grates, slices, and chops foods while shooting them out.

If you are going to be eating more vegetables and fruits, you must have *sharp knives* and a *cutting board*. There are now cutting boards made of durable plastic. These are more sanitary than wood and can be washed in the dishwasher.

Substitutes

There are some items available that help you get the flavor and cooking effect you want without adding more fat. For example, use cooking spray and butter-flavored flakes instead of oil or butter. Add these kinds of substitutes to your kitchen repertoire.

Personal Evaluation

- Which of these items are missing from your kitchen?
- Which of these might help you cook and eat in less fattening ways?
- If you don't have extra money in your budget now, are you willing to plan these items into your budget?

Action

1. Clean out your pantry, eliminating the foods that are high-fat and high in refined sugars, plus other foods you think contribute to your being overweight.
2. Purchase or plan to purchase as many of these items as you think will be helpful to you.

Encouragement

When you redesign your kitchen to match your new focus on healthy eating, you will help yourself lose weight.

DAY

18

Planning to Eat Out

Having a strategy for eating out is necessary to help you lose weight and keep it off. You probably eat out at restaurants and fast-food establishments from time to time. You may even eat out more than you eat at home. Whatever the frequency, some preplanning concerning eating out will help you.

———————•———————

You don't have to feel deprived when eating out.

As you read through the following suggestions, consider what kinds of changes you could make that would still be enjoyable for you. If you make choices that leave you feeling deprived, especially when you are out with a group of friends or celebrating a special occasion, you will not continue with them.

Find Some New Places You Like to Eat

Don't stay in the same old rut; look for new places to eat out. Some of these will have great food that isn't as fattening as what you are used to eating. Check advertisements in the entertainment section of the paper, in health-food establishments, and in your yellow pages. This would be a good time to find restaurants you like that feature dishes relying primarily on grains and vegetables, such as Thai, Chinese, Japanese, and other restaurants serving international cuisine. There are even some restaurants that focus their entire menu on low-fat, nutritious options. Keep trying new places until you find a few you enjoy.

Try Some New Menu Items That Are Less Fattening

Even at the restaurants you already frequent, you should be able to find new menu items that aren't as fattening. When you find alternatives to high-fat previous favorites, order those at least half the time. Many restaurants are becoming more health and fat conscious. In response to consumer demand, they may have a list of lighter meals on the menu. If they don't, you can still ask the server to suggest something from the menu that is tasty and yet not fattening.

Get Nutritional Information for Fast Food

Fast-food restaurants have nutritional information available for the asking. This will tell you the ingredients used in each menu item and other information, such as amount of fat, calories, and so on. Identify which menu items would be healthier choices, and order these every other time you visit. You may find something you like more than what you used to order. In this case, you can make the switch permanent. Either way is an improvement.

Consider Your Old Favorites, Cooked a Less Fattening Way

The way foods are cooked has a lot to do with the amount of fat you consume. Become aware of how many fried foods you eat, since these are very high in fat. Look for new ways of having the same food prepared; it can still taste good. If you are used to eating poultry with the skin, you are eating a lot of fat (contained in the skin). Ask to have poultry cooked without the skin if possible, or choose a skinless option. Even some fast food restaurants offer skin-free chicken. It tastes almost as though it has the skin on because of the spices used. Try to discover what preparation options are available in certain restaurants. They may be willing to prepare your food in less fattening ways, such as broiling (without butter), boiling, steaming, poaching, or baking.

Plan for Dessert Ahead of Time

The type of restaurant you choose will determine the kinds of desserts you will be faced with at the end of your meal. If you know you can't resist the house favorite, Chocolate Decadence, perhaps you should limit the number of times you must face the temptation. If you have a hard time resisting what you see, at the beginning of the meal ask the server not to bring the dessert tray to your table. If you are traveling on an airplane and want to avoid dessert, ask the flight attendant to remove the dessert from your tray before delivering it.

Try to find a dessert you can enjoy that isn't going to ruin all the good you did by eating a light meal. Look at the lighter desserts and find one you like, or share a dessert among several people.

Personal Evaluation

- What restaurants do you frequent?
- Do they have lighter fare available on the menu?
- What fried foods are a regular part of your diet? Are there other ways of cooking these foods that you might enjoy?
- Are you willing to look for new places to eat and new menu selections to help yourself lose weight?

Action

1. Do whatever research is necessary to come up with a list of restaurants that have great, nutritious food that is less fattening than what you are used to

eating. Write the names and phone numbers of these restaurants in a place where you can refer to them when necessary.

2. Since you are still eating primarily fruits, vegetables, and grain products, take this opportunity to try to find restaurants that have delicious meals using these basic foods.

3. Write out a list of menu items you usually order that could be less fattening if cooked differently. The next time you go out, try ordering the food cooked this new way.

4. Whenever you go out to eat, plan ahead to decide what strategy you are going to use to keep dessert from overwhelming your good intention. Write down three ways you could (and would be willing to) do dessert differently that would be less fattening than your old habits.

Encouragement

You don't need to give up eating out and enjoying social times centered around food. By preparing to eat out healthfully, you can still lose weight without missing out on all the fun.

DAY
19

Rediscovering Dairy Foods

By now you are probably missing your favorite dairy foods and are ready to bring them back into your life. For many people, the dairy case becomes a treasure trove of tasty, fattening foods. Dairy products bring a richness to foods—and often bring that rich flavor in the form of fat. Just think of all the great foods that fall into this category: butter, sour cream, cream cheese, whipped cream, milk, a wide assortment of cheeses, yogurt, puddings . . . and the list goes on. Today you are going to rediscover dairy foods.

●

Rediscover dairy foods.

Recall one of the reasons for your taking some time out from eating the way you used to: to give yourself a better chance of appreciating some of the low-fat and fat-free alternatives now available. Since you haven't been eating your favorite dairy products for several days, you may be more open to trying low-fat substitutes for your old high-fat favorites.

You may not have noticed, but there are low-fat and fat-free alternatives for almost every kind of food in the dairy case. Some examples are fat-free cream cheese, low-fat yogurt, light (2 percent fat) and extra-light (1 percent fat) milk, nonfat milk, reduced-fat cheeses, ice milk, non-fat frozen yogurt, and the like. Today you are going to rediscover the dairy case by trying some low-fat and fat-free products that are substitutes for your old favorites.

No one is going to force you to eat these things for the rest of your life. That is not the point of this exercise. Instead, you will want to discover which of these fat savers you really like, which taste good enough to encourage you to lose the fat and keep the flavor, and which can be substituted in your cooking without losing the richness of flavor they bring to your food. One thing to be aware of is that even though margarine may have fewer grams of fat than butter, 90 percent to 100 percent of calories still come from fat.

You are looking for substitutes that let you enjoy

the same kind of eating experience with less fattening effect. For example, if you have been in the habit of having toast with butter, jam, and/or cream cheese, you would significantly reduce the fat if you found a whole-grain bagel you enjoyed with fat-free cream cheese (which really tastes almost the same as regular cream cheese) and/or spreadable fruit (puréed fruit without any added sugar).

You don't have to give up the taste of dairy foods you love to lose weight. You don't have to force yourself to eat only low-fat cottage cheese. You can now find plenty of good-tasting, less fattening alternatives. Remember, you are trying to make changes that will be improvements over the way you used to eat, without your losing the enjoyment of eating. Therefore, if you focus on the foods you like and find reduced-fat alternatives, you will have a much more enjoyable and successful weight-loss experience.

Personal Evaluation

- What dairy foods have you been missing that you look forward to reincorporating in your diet?
- Are you willing to try only low-fat and fat-free alternatives on this shopping trip so you can discover a few alternatives you really enjoy?

Action

1. Use the menu and shopping list you prepared on day 16. Determine to buy only the food items on

your list, along with those that fit with today's action plan.

2. Be sure to eat a satisfying meal (of fruits, grains, and vegetables) before you go to the store.

3. You may want to help yourself notice new alternatives by shopping at a store other than the one you usually patronize. If you go to your familiar market, it will be more difficult to keep from gravitating toward the items you used to buy.

4. Go on a fat-free, low-fat scavenger hunt. Search the dairy case, the salad dressing aisle, and anywhere you might find fat-free alternatives to old favorites. Only buy items that are fat free or have less than 25 percent of calories from fat. Later you can choose which ones to stay with and which old favorites you want to use in moderation.

5. When you get home from the store, prepare your vegetables for healthy, handy snacks. Fix yourself a "treat," using your new alternate dairy items.

Encouragement

If you can find foods that taste as good as old favorites with less fattening effect, you won't have to give up the tastes you love in order to lose the fat you don't want.

The human body is designed to tell you what you need to eat. People low in potassium may crave bananas, which are rich in potassium. Pregnant women are renowned for their cravings. These cravings often give the woman insight into which foods will satisfy the nutritional needs of her developing baby and her rapidly changing body. You don't need a degree in nutrition to learn to eat healthfully. If you begin to eat nutritious foods in their unprocessed state, you will become more sensitive to the kinds of food your body needs to stay healthy and at a healthy weight.

Many people assume they will never be able to eat the things they crave. They are perpetually fighting off their body's hunger signals and confusing the body by eating processed foods that are high in refined sugars and other stimulants. If you give yourself the chance to stop dieting and start eating a healthy, low-fat diet, you will have the opportunity to eat whatever you want. If you are truly listening to your body's hunger signals, you will want healthy foods.

———————•———————

Listen to your body's hunger signals for healthy foods.

———————————

One woman I know is living proof of this. She always thought she would gravitate toward sweets if she allowed herself to listen to her body. She had been on and off diets for several years, weighing 170 pounds at a height of 5′2″. Her cycle was to diet vigorously, lose some weight, then give in to her craving for sweets and binge on every kind of dessert and candy she could reach.

Finally she decided to stop trying to lose weight (after a nineteen-day juice fast) and consulted a nutritionist. Her new goal became to eat a healthy, balanced diet and to resist being so compulsive in response to her "sweet tooth." The doctor "prescribed" a healthy variety of unprocessed foods: fruits, vegetables, whole grains, moderate amounts of dairy products, fish, poultry, and sparing use of red meat. He told her to eliminate all white sugar, other forms of processed sugar, and processed foods. She kept on the program well because she had had so much practice with dieting. The doctor further encouraged her to listen to her body and eat whatever good foods she craved until she was no longer hungry.

After a few months, she was amazed to find that her old cravings for sweets did not plague her. Within a year she had lost forty pounds and had no cravings for sweets. Several years have now passed. She is no longer so restrictive in her choice of foods and will, on occasion, eat desserts prepared with copious amounts of fat, sugar, and chocolate (her old nemesis). She is amazed that often she will eat a few bites and not want any more. She lives at a normal weight, eats whenever she is hungry, and finds that her body is her friend. She has learned to trust her body to tell her which good foods to eat.

Your body wants to help you lose weight and stay in shape. You too can learn to listen to what your body is telling you. Following are some suggestions to help you stay in tune with your body and its needs.

Ask Yourself What You Are Hungry For

When you think you are feeling hungry, focus your attention on your body and how it feels. Don't expose yourself to food you can see; the visual stimulation may cause you to become distracted. Instead, go through a list of good foods in your mind. Do you want bread? cereal? an apple? fish? a sandwich? a salad? a bagel and cream cheese (fat free, of course)? When something sounds good, decide exactly what you will eat before going to get it from your kitchen or a restaurant.

Stop Eating If What You Have Doesn't Hit the Spot

If you are eating something and it doesn't seem to satisfy what your body is hungry for, stop eating for the sake of eating. This is not to say that you reject food at each meal. You will need a balance of healthy foods, and your meals should be planned to supply them. However, if you are hungry between meals, don't force yourself to eat all of something if it isn't satisfying. Get in the habit of saving food for another time instead of eating the whole thing because it is there.

If you still want something but you're not sure what, have a drink of water. Then try something else.

Start with Natural Foods

If you are craving something sweet, try eating a piece of fruit before a candy bar. You may still decide to go with the candy bar later, but many times the fruit will satisfy you. Then the candy bar isn't as alluring.

Personal Evaluation

- Can you remember a time when you were able to hear your body's cravings for specific foods you needed at the time?
- Are you willing to explore the possibility that your body can direct you to the kinds of foods you need without causing you to stay fat?
- Will you try the aforementioned strategies to

learn to listen to your body? Doing so can help you every time you feel hungry.

Action

1. Continue listening to your body's hunger signals. Then eat in response to those hunger signals rather than eating continuously.
2. For the remainder of your thirty days, whenever you feel hungry take a moment to ask yourself what you are hungry for before deciding what you will eat.
3. If you are following your menu plan and find yourself craving a different kind of food than you have planned, allow yourself the flexibility to move meals around within your plan or to make healthy substitutions.

Encouragement

It is incredibly freeing to be able to trust your body to guide you to the foods you need. Give yourself the chance to experience this freedom.

21

Picking Up the Pace

As part of your new daily routine, by now you should be physically moving somewhat more than you were before. I hope you are enjoying the boost in energy from taking recess and walking or doing other small things that increase your overall activity level. However, now it is time to pick up the pace a bit.

Exercise is a great boost to weight loss because it not only helps burn energy (stored in fat), but also can increase your metabolism rate so that fat is burned more quickly. If you rely on dieting alone to lose weight (without exercise), you will be fighting an uphill battle. A restrictive diet will cause your body to conserve energy (stored as fat) by reducing the metabolism rate at which your body burns fat. Therefore, to maximize your weight-loss efforts, you need to find an exercise activity that will elevate your pulse rate and keep it at an aerobic level for at least twenty minutes, three or four times each week.

————————●————————

Find a safe, effective way to exercise.

If you are out of shape because you have not exercised regularly for a long time, find something you can do without injury or muscle strain. It is good to start with activities that have low impact, such as swimming, low-impact aerobics, or roller-skating. These activities do not jar the body as running would. It is always a good idea to consult a health-care professional who knows your medical history to advise you on which exercise activities would be safe and effective for you.

There are many exercise videos at various levels of exertion, aimed at various age levels and using a wide range of accompanying music. Start where you are. To find an exercise video you will use, rent various ones from your local video store before choosing to purchase one.

Personal Evaluation

- Can you think of any kind of physical activity you have enjoyed at some time in your life?
- Which members of your family might be willing to start an exercise commitment with you?
- Would you prefer exercising in the privacy of your home or with others? Can you think of people with whom you could exercise?
- Are you willing to try exercising four times a week (twenty-minute sessions) for the next two months before deciding to give it up?
- What time of day do you feel the most energetic? How could you arrange to use this time of day to exercise?

Action

1. Make a commitment to explore various activities that you might enjoy enough to continue exercising on a regular basis.
2. Make sure you have enough time in your schedule to accommodate four twenty-minute exercise sessions each week.
3. Consider the following list of activities, and circle any that interest you as a form of aerobic exercise. Also list any other exercise options you enjoy.

dance class	aerobics class	basketball
treadmill	rowing	running/
exercise video	machine	jogging
stair climbing	swimming	skiing machine
volleyball	bicycling	jumping rope

racquetball	skiing	tennis
soccer	hiking	calisthenics
skating		

4. Select or purchase an outfit of clothing to use when you exercise. This will help you get moving in the right direction. Since this exercise routine is new for you, you will probably encounter some internal resistance when you begin. You won't feel like exercising until you get used to it. However, once you get your body moving, the effects of the activity will probably help you feel more positive about what you are doing. Therefore, just tell yourself to start by changing into your exercise clothes.
5. Decide what you will do and when you will do it. Write this commitment in your schedule.
6. If it will help you, find a friend or family member to agree to exercise with you for the next two months. Then encourage each other.
7. Within three days, start your exercise routine at the new pace. Continue the other routines that you began on day 9.

Encouragement

Be careful not to demand too much of yourself in the beginning. Instead, applaud whatever progress you make from the level of exercise you previously had.

Eliminating Exercise Excuses

If you don't exercise on a regular basis, you probably have a few good reasons. Some people might call them excuses. Whatever they are called, unless you face them honestly and get around them, you probably won't change your life enough to maintain the weight loss you desire.

———————●———————

You can overcome your exercise excuses.

There are probably more good reasons for overcoming your objections to exercising than there are reasons not to exercise. Following are some of them.

Health Reasons

If you believe you can't exercise because of health problems, the truth may be that exercise is part of the solution to your health problems. Your lack of exercise may be a major contributing factor to your poor health. Exercise strengthens and stretches your body. Your doctor can advise you of some exercise you can do.

Improved Sex Life

For the sake of your sex life alone, there is plenty of motivation to get you moving. A recent article in a popular magazine noted that moderate exercise one hour a day, three times a week can have a dramatic effect on a marriage. Several research studies noted in the article showed that people who exercised regularly experience physiological changes that create a "sexual second wind," have more stamina, more easily ward off the blues by releasing endorphins (mood-elevating hormones) into the bloodstream, develop a better self-image, experience a significant jump in sexual confidence, feel more attractive, and have an increase in sexual desire and satisfaction after several months of exercising.

Stress Reduction

Stress is a major factor in modern life and contributes heavily to physical and emotional ailments. Exer-

cise can be used to help you burn off stress and eliminate the physical results of stress in your body.

Improved Appearance and Self-Esteem

When you exercise regularly for a period of time,
you will gain a sense of accomplishment for doing
something that is so worthwhile for your body. Your
physical appearance can't help but improve. Your im-
proved appearance will be an added boost to your
self-esteem.

More Energy

You will find that regular exercise will not wear
you out. In fact, you should experience having more
energy than you did when you were not exercising.
Many people who thought they were too tired to exercise are amazed that their fatigue disappears when
they maintain a regular exercise program.

The Overcoming of an Aversion to Exercise

Even though there are obvious benefits to exercising, you may be a person who has an aversion to exercise for more emotional reasons. Many people who
have lived in overweight bodies in a weight-conscious
society have this aversion. However, you can find
some form of exercise that allows you to avoid the
negative elements of the experience.

For example, one overweight woman had terrible
memories of being fat in high school. Gym class was
an exercise in humiliation; she was teased and always
picked last for team games. This woman, as an adult,

could not bring herself to participate in any exercise where she had to be around other people. What worked for her was to use Richard Simmons' "Sweatin' to the Oldies" exercise video alone in her home. This tape shows men and women of various shapes and sizes (many far heavier than she was). Therefore, she did not feel humiliated comparing herself to thin persons, as she had in high school.

Personal Evaluation

- Are there health reasons that prevent you from exercising?
- Are there practical reasons why you do not exercise?
- If you don't like to exercise, what are the emotional reasons for this aversion?
- What past experiences may cause you to shy away from an exercise program?

Action

1. If you can identify the obstacles that keep you from exercising, you will be able to find some way to get around each particular obstacle. Therefore, give consideration to the real reason you avoid exercising. In your notebook, divide a sheet of paper into two columns.
2. In the lefthand column list the following:

   - All the health-related reasons you have for not exercising regularly.

- All the practical reasons you have for not exercising regularly. Include scheduling, family and work-related obligations, lack of appropriate clothing, and so on.
- All the emotional reasons you have for not exercising.

3. In the righthand column list ways you could work to get around each obstacle.
4. Describe any emotional aversion you feel when you think of exercising (either to your support person or in writing). If you find that you cannot get beyond these emotional roadblocks on your own, consider seeking the help of a professional therapist.

Encouragement

Even if you have many obstacles that discourage you from exercising regularly, you can overcome them. Encourage yourself to deal with each one individually so that you can enjoy the benefits exercise will bring you.

Food for Thought

We should not let our fears hold us back from pursuing our hopes.

—John F. Kennedy

Old Messages and
Your New Life

When you learn to live a new lifestyle, you will also need to challenge the old messages still rattling around in your mind. Your tendency to stay overweight is related to life patterns and life choices influenced by the way you think. In order to maintain a new, lighter weight and lifestyle, you will need to practice thinking in new ways.

Only you know the particular messages spoken about you by others or the things you say to yourself that influence your actions. You need to identify any old messages that are counterproductive to your new lifestyle. Then you can recognize and correct them when they threaten to trigger old ways of life.

Following are examples of some ways old mental

tapes can sabotage your success. These may not be the same negative messages as those you have in your mind. However, you will be able to identify your own as you focus your attention in this direction.

Negative Self-Talk

Examples are statements such as, "I might as well give up. No matter what I do, I can't keep the weight off." These statements may or may not be true of your past, but you can change. They are not necessarily true of your future.

"She's Our Pleasingly Plump Child"

Some families have a need to have a "plump" child. There has been much written in recent years about family systems that become rigid, demanding that each person play a particular role in the family. Dysfunctional families may be threatened when someone starts to change for the better. Don't let family members' designation of you as the "plump one" or "fat one" keep you living in an overweight body.

Irrational Guilt Trips

"Clean your plate! There are children starving in China." This familiar phrase and others like it have become the motivation for many to overeat at every meal. Although it is true and very sad that children are starving in China and even in America, your over-eating doesn't help them one little bit. The next time you are about to eat food you are not hungry for, in response to messages like this, don't do it. Instead, you may want to choose to do something that relieves your guilt and actually helps starving children. Perhaps you could keep a small bank on your table. Every time you stop eating without cleaning your plate, make a donation. At the end of each month, send the money to a charitable organization that feeds starving children.

---●---

***Send money, not worthless
good intentions, to the starving
children!***

"*I Paid for It; I Should Eat It*"

You may find that when you pay good money for a meal at a restaurant, you can't bring yourself to leave any food uneaten. Learn to deal with this in a new way. You can bring the food home and eat it later. Or try this instead: tell yourself that you bought the privilege of choosing how much to eat and how much to leave on your plate. The fact that you purchased a meal (which may be oversized) is no reason to force yourself to weigh more than you want to.

Perception of Yourself As a Person on a Restrictive Diet

Don't let yourself stay in the deprivation mode. You can have foods you want—even some that are fattening—as long as your general eating patterns are changed to help you maintain a healthy weight. Remind yourself of all the good foods you are giving your body instead of focusing on the foods and ways of eating you are choosing to change.

Personal Evaluation

- What are the old messages that influence the way you tend to eat, live, and relate to food?
- Are you willing to change the old messages in order to maintain your new lifestyle?

Action

1. In your notebook, list all the old messages that could negatively influence your new lifestyle.
2. After each one, list the new way you will respond to the old message in order to enjoy your new life.

Encouragement

You can change your mind and, in so doing, change your life and your body.

Food for Thought

You are where you are, you are what you are because of what has gone into your mind. You can change where you are and what you are by changing what goes into your mind.

—Zig Ziglar

Bringing Back Meats and Fish

Today you will reintroduce meats, poultry, and fish into your life. Perhaps you are amazed that you were able to satisfy your hunger without eating meat. Hopefully, this experience will allow you to become more comfortable with keeping the amount of meat you eat at around six ounces. The recommended daily serving is about the size of two decks of playing cards. Most Americans eat more than that on a daily basis.

Following are some suggestions to keep in mind when reintroducing meats into your daily routine.

- Take advantage of this unique experience, which has already prepared you to appreciate six ounces of meat, poultry, or fish each day. Instead of overdoing it with meat that you've been missing, try to eat a balance of foods as they are recommended on the pyramid from day 5.

- Reduce the amount of red meat you eat by including less fattening meats, such as turkey and chicken, more often in your meals.
- Choose cuts of meat that have less fat. The labels on most cuts of packaged beef will tell you the percentage of fat. Try to keep the percentage as low as possible, at least under 30 percent.
- Mix meats to get flavor with less fat. If you like the flavor of ground beef and don't want to switch to ground turkey, try a mixture. Select ground beef that is low in fat, but use only half as much. Mix this with ground turkey in dishes for which you previously would have used all ground beef.
- Trim fat from meat before cooking. If you buy meat from a butcher, ask the butcher to remove the fat. Or cut it off yourself before cooking.
- Remove skin from poultry. If possible, remove skin from poultry before cooking. If that is not an option, remove the skin before eating.
- Try a new cookbook. You will have an easier time creating reduced-fat meals that use meat if you have new ideas.
- Spread your meat around. Get in the habit of making your meat go farther. Instead of serving meat as the main dish, slice it and spread it around in a dish largely consisting of vegetables, pastas, or grains.
- Don't have meat at every meal or every day.

Personal Evaluation

Are you willing to try some of these new strategies for using meat in the recommended amount?

Action

1. Plan menus for the next six days, as close as you can get to meeting the recommendations on the pyramid. Make your shopping list from this collection of menus, and eat a healthy meal before you shop.
2. Begin by selecting your fruits, vegetables, and produce. Then shop for frozen and canned goods. Next choose grains, cereals, and pastas, leaving your meats for last. There is something about having a cart that is already full of good food that can encourage you to be sensible when choosing your meats.
3. As when you chose your dairy products before, select low-fat and fat-free alternatives.
4. Choose low-fat meat options. Be sure to include some ground turkey to mix with ground beef.
5. When you get home, remember to prepare your fruits and vegetables to have available for snacks.

Encouragement

Enjoy this chance to see how your body can feel when you are eating a healthy selection of foods in their appropriate proportions.

DAY

25

Revising Old Favorites

On day 13 you made a list of ten of your favorite meals to cook or eat. Today you will revise your old favorites in ways that allow you to have those meals in a less fattening way. Each person will have a different list to revise, but the changes you can make will be similar.

Review all the new foods you have tried. Consider the ways you have discovered to reduce fat in the foods you eat without losing the flavor. Then use your own creativity to make decisions on how to adapt your old favorite recipes. Following are some general ways you can reduce the fattening effects by revision.

- Change the ingredients to low-fat or fat-free substitutes
- Add new foods that are filling and rich in fiber
- Reduce the amount of meat used and the amount of fat in the meat
- Change your cooking methods
- Spice the recipe up by using herbs and spices rather than high-fat or high-sugar ingredients

As an example of how to revise a recipe, let's say your old favorite was homemade tacos. You used to use corn tortillas, fried in a skillet, filled with ground beef, then served topped with grated cheese and sour cream.

You could make a big difference in the fat content (without losing the flavor) by making the following simple changes.

1. Instead of frying the tortillas, hang them over the wires in the oven and bake them.
2. For the meat filling, use a mixture of half ground beef with only 15 percent fat and half ground turkey, seasoned with your favorite spices.
3. Use grated low-fat or fat-free cheese.
4. Use low-fat sour cream.
5. Use plenty of lettuce, tomato, and chopped cilantro to add extra zest.

Personal Evaluation

Are you willing to at least try each of your old favorites in a revised, less fattening edition?

Action

1. In your notebook, refer back to your list of old favorites from day 13. Choose one.
2. Write out a revised recipe and cooking procedure that would make your old favorite less fattening but still as tasty.
3. Keep this list, and plan to try your revised recipe the next time you cook this dish or have it cooked for you. Note each time you actually try your new way of preparing your old favorite. Consider if what you gain in healthfulness is warranted by the taste.

Encouragement

When you choose to change the way you prepare old favorites, you won't have to give up that which is familiar to maintain your new weight.

"Good" Days and "Bad" Days

If you have tried dieting, you have also had the experience of "falling off your diet." For many people, the experience of falling off a restrictive diet triggers a chain of reactions that can be disastrous to your health. The typical scenario goes something like this:

1. You decide to finally face the fact that you are overweight and determine to lose weight—right away.
2. You endure a restrictive diet until you succumb to temptation and eat something you are not supposed to have.
3. Your momentary enjoyment of the food is quickly replaced by guilt and self-condemnation.

4. You may give in to the belief that every time you have tried to diet, you have failed. Therefore, you are destined to be overweight.
5. Since you are going to be overweight anyway, you might as well revert to your old eating patterns and give up on your latest diet.
6. You proceed in this way until you have regained the weight you lost on the diet (and perhaps more). Then you finally find yourself back at 1. You determine to lose weight again.

Going up and down in weight (gaining and losing ten or more pounds regularly) as a pattern of life is damaging to your health. You need to break this pattern. Lose ten pounds and keep them off. One of the keys to breaking the cycle is to learn to think of the "good" and "bad" days in a new way.

———————●———————

Break the pattern of fluctuating weight as a way of life.

In your new way of thinking, you will learn to see your health and weight maintenance as a long-term, ongoing goal that is reached by making a transition into a new way of living and eating. It is not some desperate measure you take before your high school reunion, only to be put aside once that special event has passed. To help you maintain this perspective, keep a running record of your weight, checking it once each week at the most. This will give you a sense of progress that doesn't depress you every day you happen to go up or stay the same.

There will be weeks when your body may gain some weight or stay the same, even if you continue to make healthy choices about your eating and activity level. This is normal and should be accepted. As long as you are moving in the right direction or staying in a healthy weight range, you need not despair.

---------------•---------------

To indulge yourself is not to have a "bad" day.

When you are living within a typical dieting cycle, the "good" days occur when you stay on your diet. The "bad" days occur when you eat one of the foods overweight people are not supposed to eat (to your old way of thinking). In your new way of thinking, accept that there are days and events when you can allow yourself to eat foods that would be fattening if eaten on a regular basis. Since you have not been starving yourself, your cravings should not be overwhelming.

A day when you allow yourself to eat foods that are an indulgence is not a bad day. It can be a good day too—a day you can enjoy a treat without triggering the despair that can cause you to become totally irresponsible about healthy eating choices. All you need to balance these days is to maintain a generally less fattening lifestyle (which you will design for yourself before this adventure ends) and perhaps to give yourself a few light days following a day of indulgence.

Remember that it takes 3,500 calories to make one pound of fat in your body. You can use this realization to encourage you. Even if you were indulgent and ate something you knew was loaded with calories from fat and high in refined sugars, so what? If this was an out-of-the-ordinary occurrence, that incident probably didn't amount to more than 3,500 calories. Just tell yourself that you can easily compensate for this allowance. Exercise a bit longer for the next week (not as punishment for guilt but as a healthy way to help your body compensate), and stay with your new healthy lifestyle.

Studies show that if your overall diet and lifestyle is low-fat and nutritious, your body can accommodate the occasional splurge without much strain. In fact, your body has a much easier time accommodating this than living with the strain of fluctuating weight from up-and-down dieting.

Personal Evaluation

- Have you ever been caught in the cycle of yo-yo dieting described here?
- Are you willing to learn to rid your mind of your old attitudes about "good" and "bad" days to help yourself maintain a healthy weight?

Action

1. Don't weigh yourself yet, but pick a day of the week to be your regular day for weighing and recording your weight.
2. In your notebook draw a chart or graph for recording your weight from week to week, starting after you finish this adventure.
3. Write out a new definition of indulgence, or think through what it means when you do eat something indulgent. Stay away from self-condemnation (thinking of yourself as bad) and designating the whole day as a "bad" day.
4. Write a three-day plan to use as an adjustment after a day when you indulge yourself with some foods that are not the best low-fat choices.

Encouragement

When you learn to see weight maintenance as a part of your ongoing healthy lifestyle, you will be freed from the tyranny of having a "bad" day.

Discovering Your List
of Helpful Hints

As you continue to live and eat in a new way, you need to collect your own list of tips that help you. These can be aids to help you continue eating in a healthy, low-fat way, to help you think of yourself in a new way as someone who is not destined to remain overweight, or to help in the area of exercise.

If you check with people who have lost weight, gotten in shape, or dramatically changed their appearance, they will probably have a list of things that helped them make the transition. They may tell you their favorite low-calorie treats that taste like "the real thing." They may tell you about a great selection of frozen foods that they use to supplement their healthy cooking when they don't have time to cook, but want to resist eating something fattening for the sake of convenience alone. They may share their enthusiasm for a particular gym, aerobics class, or exercise video. People who have succeeded in improving their health and appearance by losing weight and keeping it off usually love to share their helpful hints.

———————————●———————————

***You may find people asking you
for helpful hints.***

———————————————————

Begin noticing who around you has maintained a healthy change or a healthy physical appearance for three months or more. Ask for their helpful hints, and note any you may want to try. This will keep you from growing bored with your new lifestyle and will help you maintain enthusiasm. You will also find that you will have some tips of your own that others will appreciate hearing. You will begin seeing yourself as "one of them," the people who take care of their health.

Personal Evaluation

- Have you discovered some helps you are using to change your life to weigh less and improve your health?
- Think of some people you know who have im-

proved their health and lost weight (and kept it
off).

• Are you willing to ask others the secrets they
have found to maintaining their healthy weight
and staying in shape?

Action

1. Review your progress so far, and make a list of all
   the aids you have found that have helped you make
   good changes in your lifestyle with regard to your
   weight and health.
2. Ask some people for their favorite healthy hints.
3. If someone tells you about the latest fad or crash
   diet, be polite but don't go back. Continue eating a
   healthy balance of foods, generally with less than
   30 percent of your calories from fat, and maintaining a regular program of physical activity.

Encouragement

You will discover those "secrets" that help you lose
weight and keep it off. When you do, people will probably start asking you how you did it. So keep your list
handy!

D A Y
28

The Choices Are
All Yours

This plan has given you a direction to follow regarding what to eat along the way. In the beginning you ate just as you had been eating previously, while taking note of what you ate and why. Then you ate primarily fruits and vegetables. Then you added grain products; next you added dairy products. Finally you reintroduced meats, poultry, and fish. You never focused on what you were not eating, but fats, oils, and sweets were not part of the program.

At each point you had an opportunity to look in a new way at the foods most overweight people don't eat enough of. You were encouraged to explore ways to enjoy the nutritious foods available that are recommended for your general health, but you had free choice within each category. Part of the exercise was to concentrate your attention on making healthy choices in each area. Now you are at a point where all the choices are yours.

———————•———————

Choose to transform your lifestyle to maintain a lesser weight.

You can choose to eat whatever you like. We are blessed to live in a country where nutritious food is plentiful. When you finish this adventure, you have many choices facing you. Your first choice is whether you will transform your lifestyle to maintain a lesser weight, or whether you will go on and off diets. If you choose to continue in a lifestyle that is generally more active and less fattening, you will be choosing foods lower in fat and refined sugar. You will be choosing to find new restaurant items, new convenience foods, new cookbooks, and new ways of eating. But you are still in control. The choices are all yours.

You may have discovered that your eating was out of control. If you have found along the way that your eating patterns are compulsive and tied into emotional patterns, you may not have the freedom you would like even to follow this plan. If this is the case, you have learned a valuable lesson. You have the choice to seek help for the emotional or psychological hunger you are faced with. You may choose to seek help through a 12-Step group such as Overeaters Anonymous, read books on the subject, or seek the help of a qualified counselor who deals with eating disorders.

You may have thought that you couldn't change, but your experience during these thirty days proves that you can. You can change your lifestyle, your favorite foods, and the way you cook. In so doing, you are choosing to weigh less than you did before.

Personal Evaluation

- Do you believe now that you can change your lifestyle and, in so doing, change your health, weight, and appearance?
- Are you willing to incorporate some of the changes from your experience with this plan into your ongoing lifestyle?
- If you suspect that your weight problem is associated with an eating disorder or compulsion, are you willing to seek help for the emotional or psychological source of the behavior?
- Are you willing to give up restrictive diets for an ongoing program of healthy exercise and nutritious, low-fat eating?

Action

1. Keep an eating record for what you eat today and tomorrow, just like the ones you kept on days 3 and 4.

2. Talk with your support person, listing the choices you are making from what you have learned.
3. Choose to continue exploring your food options by looking for other foods in your market and health-food store that meet your needs nutritionally and satisfy your tastes. Determine to try some of the various dinners, lunches, breakfasts, and desserts available from weight-conscious programs.

Encouragement

When you realize that the choices are all yours and you can make good choices with regard to your weight, you will be encouraged to continue making good choices.

Food for Thought

When you choose to exercise and eat less fattening foods today, you are choosing to weigh less tomorrow.

Customizing Your
Lifestyle Plan

The goal of this adventure was for you to find your
way to change your eating habits and lifestyle so as to
lose just ten pounds. You've had the opportunity to
consider new foods and new ways of cooking. You've
replanned your life, incorporating more activity in
your normal routines and thinking in new ways. Today you will review what you have learned and expe-
rienced, then make some commitments that will help
you stay at a healthier weight.

●

Even small healthful choices can make big differences.

You don't have to do everything suggested in this book to lose weight. All you need to do is to identify where you can make less fattening choices that you can live with and change your ongoing pattern of life accordingly. Even choices that may seem insignificant prove to make a big difference when they are followed from day to day. Here is an example of the way a little change can make a big difference. If you regularly drink whole milk and switch to drinking 1 percent fat (extra-light) milk because you enjoy it just as much, it is estimated this change alone would cause you to lose ten pounds over the course of one year. Imagine what could happen if you found three or four similar changes you could live with without feeling deprived!

Personal Evaluation

- Review the way you used to eat when you took your evaluation on day 3, using the headings *When, What, Where, With Whom,* and *Why.*
- What patterns of unhealthy eating habits do you recognize as having contributed to your remaining overweight? Which of these are you willing to change to help yourself keep excess weight off?
- Review the original evaluation of your eating habits, monitoring what percentage of your calories

came from fat (day 4). What are you willing to do to reduce the percentage of calories from fat to under 30 percent?

- What new (nonfattening) foods did you discover that you liked well enough to incorporate into your life?
- What foods from your old favorites list (day 13) are you willing to adapt to become less fattening?
- Which of your fattening favorites do you want to keep just the way they are? Are you willing to have them less frequently?
- What fattening foods did you find you didn't particularly miss, even though you haven't been eating them?

Action

1. Review the observations you made in your notebook during this thirty-day period, and take action on the following ideas.
2. Make a list of good, nutritious foods you enjoy (that can help take the place of fattening old favorites) in each of the following categories: fruits, vegetables, grains, low-fat or fat-free dairy products.
3. List any changes you are willing to make in the way you prepare, cook, or order food to help reduce fat.
4. Write out what you are willing to do concerning routines that increase your general activity level on a daily basis (for example, continue taking recess, stairs instead of elevator, and so on).
5. Write out your plan for an ongoing exercise program:

I will exercise by (kind of activity) _____
_____ .
I will do this _____ times per week, typically on
(which days or evenings) _____ .
I plan to do this (where) _____ .
On days when the weather is bad, my alternate
exercise plan is to (what) _____ (where)
_____ .

6. Weigh yourself again, and compare this to your
weight when you began this adventure. You may
not have lost exactly ten pounds in these thirty
days; you may have lost more or less. However, if
you have made a transition to a less fattening way
of life, you can rest assured that you will lose the
weight you need to lose.

Encouragement

Your willingness to take a good look at the reasons
in your lifestyle for staying overweight and then to
make changes deserves a reward! The best reward is
the sense of self-satisfaction you have from losing
weight and knowing that you are making healthy
choices designed just for you. Congratulations!

Food for Thought

It is never too late to be what you might have been.
—George Eliot

Envisioning
Continued Success

According to the acclaimed motivational speaker Zig Ziglar, before you can reach any goal you must be able to see the reaching. In other words, at some point you must be able to envision your success before you will be able to reach the goal in reality. Envisioning your success provides internal motivation and encouragement when you feel like reverting back to your old familiar lifestyle. As long as you continue to see yourself as a fat person with fat habits, you will not be able to keep off the weight you lose.

You started this program with the goal of losing ten pounds. However, this is really a secondary goal. In order to achieve the effect of being ten pounds lighter, you need to adapt your lifestyle so that you will lose the fat in a way you can live with. The way to really succeed in losing ten pounds *permanently* is to have a new image of yourself, as a person living and enjoying a less fattening lifestyle.

———————●———————

Acquire a healthier, thinner self-image.

———————

If you have followed the suggestions given, you have probably lost weight. You may have lost less or more than ten pounds, but your changed lifestyle has had some effect on your body. However, the real key to losing and keeping off the excess weight comes from seeing yourself as someone who doesn't live and act like an overweight person anymore.

Personal Evaluation

- Take a few moments to think about each question following. Then focus your attention on the mental images about yourself that come to mind. Think of how you saw yourself when you began the journey and how you see yourself now (if there is a difference).
- What images do you have of yourself in terms of caring for your overall health?
- How do you see yourself in terms of energy level? Do you have images of yourself as fatigued,

plopped on the sofa after work, unable to drag yourself out of bed in the morning, or as an energetic person taking a daily walk or exercising in a way you enjoy?

- When you think of physical activity or exercise, do you see yourself on the sidelines, avoiding exercise, or enjoying exercise?

- When you imagine yourself in terms of appearance, do you see yourself as a fat person (who will always revert to being overweight), or do you see your excess weight as something foreign to your true self?

- When you describe yourself, what adjectives do you use—dumpy, frumpy, fat, plump, and the like, or other, more flattering descriptive terms such as glowing, healthy, bright-eyed, attractive, and so on?

- How do you think of yourself or envision yourself as an eater? Can you see yourself enjoying healthy food in moderation, or do you see yourself primarily as someone out of control in relation to food? Are the images of yourself when eating derogatory, such as raiding the refrigerator in secret, cramming food in your mouth, or always in a tug of war with food—sometimes starving, then binging?

Action

1. It takes faith to change your lifestyle for the better. Faith must be based on the truth of what is available for you but isn't yours yet. Faith involves believing in something that is not yet a reality—

and believing enough to take action on what you believe. You can now envision a new way of life and a body that is healthier and ten pounds lighter. This ability to envision your success will help you find your way to successfully reach your goal and go on living at the best weight for you.

Your action steps today are primarily in the form of the active use of your imagination. You are going to see where you are now and use your imagination to see the kind of person you can become.

2. Begin by looking at your body in a full-length mirror. You may have already noticed a difference in your appearance since thirty days ago. Notice the areas of your body where you may still have excess fat that needs to go. Then close your eyes and imagine what your body will look like when you lose the excess weight.

3. You may want to rely on memories of yourself when you were thinner. You may want to find a picture of someone in a magazine who is the same basic body type as you, but without excess fat. If possible, find something about yourself that is underdeveloped and see yourself as nourishing the healthy part of your life. In whatever way you approach this use of your imagination, find a way to get a clear image of what you want your body to look like without the extra pounds and what kind of person you want to become.

4. Sometime today, before you go to sleep tonight, use your imagination to see yourself as the following kind of person:

- someone who cares about your health
- someone who feels energetic
- someone who enjoys a particular kind of activity or exercise
- someone who is ten pounds thinner and more attractive than when you began this adventure
- someone who enjoys eating healthy, low-fat foods.

Encouragement

Learning to see yourself in new ways will open the doors for you to change your lifestyle permanently. You can maintain your weight loss and enjoy the benefits of excellent health.

Food for Thought

Our expectancies not only affect how we see reality, but also affect reality itself.

—Edward E. Jones